FREE Test Taking Tips DVD Offer

To help us better serve you, we have developed a Test Taking Tips DVD that we would like to give you for FREE. **This DVD covers world-class test taking tips that you can use to be even more successful when you are taking your test.**

All that we ask is that you email us your feedback about your study guide. Please let us know what you thought about it – whether that is good, bad or indifferent.

To get your **FREE Test Taking Tips DVD**, email freedvd@studyguideteam.com with "FREE DVD" in the subject line and the following information in the body of the email:

   a. The title of your study guide.

   b. Your product rating on a scale of 1-5, with 5 being the highest rating.

   c. Your feedback about the study guide. What did you think of it?

   d. Your full name and shipping address to send your free DVD.

If you have any questions or concerns, please don't hesitate to contact us at freedvd@studyguideteam.com.

Thanks again!

CCM Study Guide

CCM Certification Test Prep and Practice Test Questions for the Certified Case Manager Exam [4th Edition]

TPB Publishing

Written and edited by TPB Publishing.

TPB Publishing is not associated with or endorsed by any official testing organization. TPB Publishing is a publisher of unofficial educational products. All test and organization names are trademarks of their respective owners. Content in this book is included for utilitarian purposes only and does not constitute an endorsement by TPB Publishing of any particular point of view.

Interested in buying more than 10 copies of our product? Contact us about bulk discounts:
bulkorders@studyguideteam.com

ISBN 13: 9781628458671
ISBN 10: 1628458674

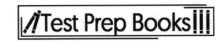

Table of Contents

Quick Overview

As you draw closer to taking your exam, effective preparation becomes more and more important. Thankfully, you have this study guide to help you get ready. Use this guide to help keep your studying on track and refer to it often.

This study guide contains several key sections that will help you be successful on your exam. The guide contains tips for what you should do the night before and the day of the test. Also included are test-taking tips. Knowing the right information is not always enough. Many well-prepared test takers struggle with exams. These tips will help equip you to accurately read, assess, and answer test questions.

A large part of the guide is devoted to showing you what content to expect on the exam and to helping you better understand that content. In this guide are practice test questions so that you can see how well you have grasped the content. Then, answer explanations are provided so that you can understand why you missed certain questions.

Don't try to cram the night before you take your exam. This is not a wise strategy for a few reasons. First, your retention of the information will be low. Your time would be better used by reviewing information you already know rather than trying to learn a lot of new information. Second, you will likely become stressed as you try to gain a large amount of knowledge in a short amount of time. Third, you will be depriving yourself of sleep. So be sure to go to bed at a reasonable time the night before. Being well-rested helps you focus and remain calm.

Be sure to eat a substantial breakfast the morning of the exam. If you are taking the exam in the afternoon, be sure to have a good lunch as well. Being hungry is distracting and can make it difficult to focus. You have hopefully spent lots of time preparing for the exam. Don't let an empty stomach get in the way of success!

When travelling to the testing center, leave earlier than needed. That way, you have a buffer in case you experience any delays. This will help you remain calm and will keep you from missing your appointment time at the testing center.

Be sure to pace yourself during the exam. Don't try to rush through the exam. There is no need to risk performing poorly on the exam just so you can leave the testing center early. Allow yourself to use all of the allotted time if needed.

Remain positive while taking the exam even if you feel like you are performing poorly. Thinking about the content you should have mastered will not help you perform better on the exam.

Once the exam is complete, take some time to relax. Even if you feel that you need to take the exam again, you will be well served by some down time before you begin studying again. It's often easier to convince yourself to study if you know that it will come with a reward!

Test-Taking Strategies

1. Predicting the Answer

When you feel confident in your preparation for a multiple-choice test, try predicting the answer before reading the answer choices. This is especially useful on questions that test objective factual knowledge. By predicting the answer before reading the available choices, you eliminate the possibility that you will be distracted or led astray by an incorrect answer choice. You will feel more confident in your selection if you read the question, predict the answer, and then find your prediction among the answer choices. After using this strategy, be sure to still read all of the answer choices carefully and completely. If you feel unprepared, you should not attempt to predict the answers. This would be a waste of time and an opportunity for your mind to wander in the wrong direction.

2. Reading the Whole Question

Too often, test takers scan a multiple-choice question, recognize a few familiar words, and immediately jump to the answer choices. Test authors are aware of this common impatience, and they will sometimes prey upon it. For instance, a test author might subtly turn the question into a negative, or he or she might redirect the focus of the question right at the end. The only way to avoid falling into these traps is to read the entirety of the question carefully before reading the answer choices.

3. Looking for Wrong Answers

Long and complicated multiple-choice questions can be intimidating. One way to simplify a difficult multiple-choice question is to eliminate all of the answer choices that are clearly wrong. In most sets of answers, there will be at least one selection that can be dismissed right away. If the test is administered on paper, the test taker could draw a line through it to indicate that it may be ignored; otherwise, the test taker will have to perform this operation mentally or on scratch paper. In either case, once the obviously incorrect answers have been eliminated, the remaining choices may be considered. Sometimes identifying the clearly wrong answers will give the test taker some information about the correct answer. For instance, if one of the remaining answer choices is a direct opposite of one of the eliminated answer choices, it may well be the correct answer. The opposite of obviously wrong is obviously right! Of course, this is not always the case. Some answers are obviously incorrect simply because they are irrelevant to the question being asked. Still, identifying and eliminating some incorrect answer choices is a good way to simplify a multiple-choice question.

4. Don't Overanalyze

Anxious test takers often overanalyze questions. When you are nervous, your brain will often run wild, causing you to make associations and discover clues that don't actually exist. If you feel that this may be a problem for you, do whatever you can to slow down during the test. Try taking a deep breath or counting to ten. As you read and consider the question, restrict yourself to the particular words used by the author. Avoid thought tangents about what the author *really* meant, or what he or she was *trying* to say. The only things that matter on a multiple-choice test are the words that are actually in the question. You must avoid reading too much into a multiple-choice question, or supposing that the writer meant something other than what he or she wrote.

5. No Need for Panic

It is wise to learn as many strategies as possible before taking a multiple-choice test, but it is likely that you will come across a few questions for which you simply don't know the answer. In this situation, avoid panicking. Because most multiple-choice tests include dozens of questions, the relative value of a single wrong answer is small. As much as possible, you should compartmentalize each question on a multiple-choice test. In other words, you should not allow your feelings about one question to affect your success on the others. When you find a question that you either don't understand or don't know how to answer, just take a deep breath and do your best. Read the entire question slowly and carefully. Try rephrasing the question a couple of different ways. Then, read all of the answer choices carefully. After eliminating obviously wrong answers, make a selection and move on to the next question.

6. Confusing Answer Choices

When working on a difficult multiple-choice question, there may be a tendency to focus on the answer choices that are the easiest to understand. Many people, whether consciously or not, gravitate to the answer choices that require the least concentration, knowledge, and memory. This is a mistake. When you come across an answer choice that is confusing, you should give it extra attention. A question might be confusing because you do not know the subject matter to which it refers. If this is the case, don't eliminate the answer before you have affirmatively settled on another. When you come across an answer choice of this type, set it aside as you look at the remaining choices. If you can confidently assert that one of the other choices is correct, you can leave the confusing answer aside. Otherwise, you will need to take a moment to try to better understand the confusing answer choice. Rephrasing is one way to tease out the sense of a confusing answer choice.

7. Your First Instinct

Many people struggle with multiple-choice tests because they overthink the questions. If you have studied sufficiently for the test, you should be prepared to trust your first instinct once you have carefully and completely read the question and all of the answer choices. There is a great deal of research suggesting that the mind can come to the correct conclusion very quickly once it has obtained all of the relevant information. At times, it may seem to you as if your intuition is working faster even than your reasoning mind. This may in fact be true. The knowledge you obtain while studying may be retrieved from your subconscious before you have a chance to work out the associations that support it. Verify your instinct by working out the reasons that it should be trusted.

8. Key Words

Many test takers struggle with multiple-choice questions because they have poor reading comprehension skills. Quickly reading and understanding a multiple-choice question requires a mixture of skill and experience. To help with this, try jotting down a few key words and phrases on a piece of scrap paper. Doing this concentrates the process of reading and forces the mind to weigh the relative importance of the question's parts. In selecting words and phrases to write down, the test taker thinks about the question more deeply and carefully. This is especially true for multiple-choice questions that are preceded by a long prompt.

9. Subtle Negatives

One of the oldest tricks in the multiple-choice test writer's book is to subtly reverse the meaning of a question with a word like *not* or *except*. If you are not paying attention to each word in the question, you can easily be led astray by this trick. For instance, a common question format is, "Which of the following is…?" Obviously, if the question instead is, "Which of the following is not…?," then the answer will be quite different. Even worse, the test makers are aware of the potential for this mistake and will include one answer choice that would be correct if the question were not negated or reversed. A test taker who misses the reversal will find what he or she believes to be a correct answer and will be so confident that he or she will fail to reread the question and discover the original error. The only way to avoid this is to practice a wide variety of multiple-choice questions and to pay close attention to each and every word.

10. Reading Every Answer Choice

It may seem obvious, but you should always read every one of the answer choices! Too many test takers fall into the habit of scanning the question and assuming that they understand the question because they recognize a few key words. From there, they pick the first answer choice that answers the question they believe they have read. Test takers who read all of the answer choices might discover that one of the latter answer choices is actually *more* correct. Moreover, reading all of the answer choices can remind you of facts related to the question that can help you arrive at the correct answer. Sometimes, a misstatement or incorrect detail in one of the latter answer choices will trigger your memory of the subject and will enable you to find the right answer. Failing to read all of the answer choices is like not reading all of the items on a restaurant menu: you might miss out on the perfect choice.

11. Spot the Hedges

One of the keys to success on multiple-choice tests is paying close attention to every word. This is never truer than with words like almost, most, some, and sometimes. These words are called "hedges" because they indicate that a statement is not totally true or not true in every place and time. An absolute statement will contain no hedges, but in many subjects, the answers are not always straightforward or absolute. There are always exceptions to the rules in these subjects. For this reason, you should favor those multiple-choice questions that contain hedging language. The presence of qualifying words indicates that the author is taking special care with his or her words, which is certainly important when composing the right answer. After all, there are many ways to be wrong, but there is only one way to be right! For this reason, it is wise to avoid answers that are absolute when taking a multiple-choice test. An absolute answer is one that says things are either all one way or all another. They often include words like *every*, *always*, *best*, and *never*. If you are taking a multiple-choice test in a subject that doesn't lend itself to absolute answers, be on your guard if you see any of these words.

12. Long Answers

In many subject areas, the answers are not simple. As already mentioned, the right answer often requires hedges. Another common feature of the answers to a complex or subjective question are qualifying clauses, which are groups of words that subtly modify the meaning of the sentence. If the question or answer choice describes a rule to which there are exceptions or the subject matter is complicated, ambiguous, or confusing, the correct answer will require many words in order to be expressed clearly and accurately. In essence, you should not be deterred by answer choices that seem excessively long. Oftentimes, the author of the text will not be able to write the correct answer without offering some qualifications and modifications. Your job is to read the answer choices thoroughly and completely and to select the one that most accurately and precisely answers the question.

13. Restating to Understand

Sometimes, a question on a multiple-choice test is difficult not because of what it asks but because of how it is written. If this is the case, restate the question or answer choice in different words. This process serves a couple of important purposes. First, it forces you to concentrate on the core of the question. In order to rephrase the question accurately, you have to understand it well. Rephrasing the question will concentrate your mind on the key words and ideas. Second, it will present the information to your mind in a fresh way. This process may trigger your memory and render some useful scrap of information picked up while studying.

14. True Statements

Sometimes an answer choice will be true in itself, but it does not answer the question. This is one of the main reasons why it is essential to read the question carefully and completely before proceeding to the answer choices. Too often, test takers skip ahead to the answer choices and look for true statements. Having found one of these, they are content to select it without reference to the question above. Obviously, this provides an easy way for test makers to play tricks. The savvy test taker will always read the entire question before turning to the answer choices. Then, having settled on a correct answer choice, he or she will refer to the original question and ensure that the selected answer is relevant. The mistake of choosing a correct-but-irrelevant answer choice is especially common on questions related to specific pieces of objective knowledge. A prepared test taker will have a wealth of factual knowledge at his or her disposal, and should not be careless in its application.

15. No Patterns

One of the more dangerous ideas that circulates about multiple-choice tests is that the correct answers tend to fall into patterns. These erroneous ideas range from a belief that B and C are the most common right answers, to the idea that an unprepared test-taker should answer "A-B-A-C-A-D-A-B-A." It cannot be emphasized enough that pattern-seeking of this type is exactly the WRONG way to approach a multiple-choice test. To begin with, it is highly unlikely that the test maker will plot the correct answers according to some predetermined pattern. The questions are scrambled and delivered in a random order. Furthermore, even if the test maker was following a pattern in the assignation of correct answers, there is no reason why the test taker would know which pattern he or she was using. Any attempt to discern a pattern in the answer choices is a waste of time and a distraction from the real work of taking the test. A test taker would be much better served by extra preparation before the test than by reliance on a pattern in the answers.

FREE DVD OFFER

Don't forget that doing well on your exam includes both understanding the test content and understanding how to use what you know to do well on the test. We offer a completely FREE Test Taking Tips DVD that covers world class test taking tips that you can use to be even more successful when you are taking your test.

All that we ask is that you email us your feedback about your study guide. To get your **FREE Test Taking Tips DVD**, email freedvd@studyguideteam.com with "FREE DVD" in the subject line and the following information in the body of the email:

- The title of your study guide.
- Your product rating on a scale of 1-5, with 5 being the highest rating.
- Your feedback about the study guide. What did you think of it?
- Your full name and shipping address to send your free DVD.

Introduction to the CCM Exam

Function of the Test

The Certified Case Manager (CCM) exam is part of the Commission for Case Manager Certification's (CCMC's) certification process. CCMC is the largest case management certification program in the United States, and touts over 60,000 case managers certified under its auspices. CCMC encourages case managers to get CCMC certification in order to gain access to jobs with employers that require certification for case managers, and to gain access to promotions and pay raises from employers who prefer such certification.

CCMC requires that individuals taking the CCM exam have at least twelve months of full-time case management experience while supervised by a certified case manager, or twenty-four months of full-time case management experience without such supervision. Accordingly, individuals who take the CCM exam are adults who are already working in the case management profession. Most have bachelor and/or graduate degrees in social work, nursing, or another health and human services field. Some employers reimburse the cost of case management continuing education for the purpose of preparing for the CCM exam.

Test Administration

Prospective test takers must apply to take the test and submit an application fee. If and when their application is approved, they must then pay a test fee to take the exam. The exam may be taken three months out of the year—April, August, and December—with applications needing to be submitted at least five months before the test date.

The test may be taken at hundreds of Prometric test centers across the United States. However, it is not necessarily offered at every Prometric location, so test-takers should check to see where the closest center offering the test is located.

If a test-taker fails the exam, he or she can schedule a retake during the next testing cycle by contacting CCMC and paying a $185 retake fee. If a retake is not scheduled during the next testing cycle, the test-taker will have to re-apply and pay the full first-time application and examination fee.

Students with documented disabilities may submit requests for accommodations to CCMC. If CCMC approves accommodations, they will be arranged between the test-taker and Prometric.

Test Format

The CCM exam is delivered by computer at the Prometric testing center. It covers five major domains of "essential knowledge" for case managers. The test consists of 180 multiple-choice questions, 150 of which are official and scored, and are divided as follows:

Domain	Approx % of test	Approx # of questions
Care Delivery and Reimbursement Methods	28	42
Psychosocial Concepts and Support Systems	25	38
Quality and Outcomes Evaluation and Measurements	19	29
Rehabilitation Concepts and Strategies	11	16
Ethical, Legal, and Practice Standards	17	25

For a $30 fee, a prospective test-taker may arrange a "test drive" appointment with Prometric, for the purpose of gaining experience with the look and feel of the test and the testing center and the process of taking the test.

Scoring

Test-takers' raw scores are based simply on the number of correct answers given, with no penalty for incorrect answers or guesses. The raw scores are scaled to equalize difficulty and compared to a required passing score, which is determined based on a panel of experts' estimates of the probability that a minimally qualified candidate would have answered the questions correctly.

Immediately upon completion of the test, the test-taker will receive a pass-fail score. CCMC says this immediate score is "99% accurate," and that the official result will come four weeks after the last exam of the testing month is given. Test-takers who pass will receive a passing certificate, while those who fail will receive a detailed scoring report.

Recent/Future Developments

The content of the CCM exam was updated as of the December 2020 exam. The new content reflects changes to the profession with the tested material organized into five major domains.

Study Prep Plan for the CCM Exam

1 **Schedule** - Use one of our study schedules below or come up with one of your own.

2 **Relax -** Test anxiety can hurt even the best students. There are many ways to reduce stress. Find the one that works best for you.

3 **Excecute** - Once you have a good plan in place, be sure to stick to it

Sample Study Plans

One Week Study Schedule		
Day 1	Care Delivery and Reimbursement Methods
Day 2	Psychosocial Concepts and Support Systems
Day 3	Quality Outcomes Evaluations and Measurements
Day 4	Rehabilitation Concepts and Strategies
Day 5	Ethical, Legal, and Practice Standards
Day 6	Review Answer Explanations
Day 7	**Take Your Exam!**

Two Week Study Schedule			
Day 1	Adherence to Care Regimen	Day 8	Functional Capacity Evaluation
Day 2	Case-Management Process and Tools	Day 9	Affordable Care Act
Day 3	Behavioral Change Theories And Stages	Day 10	Risk Management
Day 4	Client Self-Care Management	Day 11	Practice Questions
Day 5	Accreditation Standards and Requirements	Day 12	Review Answers
Day 6	Healthcare Analytics	Day 13	Review Explanations
Day 7	Assistive Devices	Day 14	**Take Your Exam!**

One Month Study Schedule

Day 1	Adherence to Care Regimen	Day 11	Support Programs	Day 21	Affordable Care Act
Day 2	Case-Management Process and Tools	Day 12	Accreditation Standards and Requirements	Day 22	Case Recording
Day 3	Managed Care Concepts	Day 13	Cost-Benefit Analysis	Day 23	Ethics Related to Care Delivery
Day 4	Private Benefit Programs	Day 14	Data Interpretation and Reporting	Day 24	Risk Management
Day 5	Abuse and Neglect	Day 15	Healthcare Analytics	Day 25	Standards of Practice
Day 6	Behavioral Health Concepts	Day 16	Program Evaluation and Research Methods	Day 26	Practice Questions
Day 7	Conflict Resolution Strategies	Day 17	Types of Quality Indicators	Day 27	Practice Questions
Day 8	End-of-Life Issues	Day 18	Assistive Devices	Day 28	Review Answers
Day 9	Interpersonal Communication	Day 19	Functional Capacity Evaluation	Day 29	Review Explanations
Day 10	Interview Techniques	Day 20	Vocational and Rehabilitation Service Delivery System	Day 30	**Take Your Exam!**

Care Delivery and Reimbursement Methods

Accountable Care Organizations

Since the Affordable Care Act introduced Accountable Care Organizations (ACOs) over a decade ago, ACOs have been working to meet the healthcare industry's "Triple Aim": decreasing costs, improving patient satisfaction, and providing quality healthcare. ACOs are groups of hospitals, physicians, and other providers that work together to coordinate patient care for financial incentive. ACOs are most often able to receive their financial incentives by saving money when they are working with a large group of providers for various services that are committed to high quality healthcare.

Traditionally, under the fee-for-service model, more care provided to a patient would equal more profit by the provider, even in some cases where the care may not have been the best or most appropriate treatment. Under ACO care, earnings can be made by taking care of a population of patients preventatively, rewarding the ACO with financial incentives for keeping patients out of hospitals, and minimizing procedures, if minimum savings rate benchmarks are met. For example, most Medicare ACO benchmarks are set at about 4 percent.

Case managers working in ACOs can look for trends in the diagnosis and treatment of patients with commonly treated disease processes, and then advocate for evidenced-based protocols for treatment regarding each patient with that disease. By doing this, ACOs can make sure that quality healthcare is received and that the correct and appropriate tests and services are done for patients. Case managers can use data from these selected patient populations, including money saved and reimbursements received, to justify cost of case managers. Case managers can be an integral part of helping patients navigate their ACO network efficiently, as they help to reduce the cost of care. Tracking patients as they move between services and transitions of care can help ACOs have a holistic view of the patient and improve patient experiences.

Since their inception, the number of ACOs has grown each year, and their impact on the healthcare system a little over a decade in has already changed the traditional pay-for-service model. Case managers can add value to this new and developing model by bringing the skills they already use in other areas, including collaboration and coordination.

Adherence to Care Regimen

Adherence to care, a phrase that is sometimes confused with the term "compliance," is an essential component of case management and positive patient outcomes. Adhering to a care regimen is a collaborative effort—one that requires both the patient and the treating provider to be engaged in the process of establishing a treatment plan. This is somewhat different from that of compliance, in which the physician dictates priorities and the patient is expected to comply. **Compliance** refers to patients following the physician's orders without giving any input as it relates to their ability to adhere to the plan of care or identify their own priorities.

Adherence to care includes keeping scheduled appointments, taking medication as prescribed, and following the overall treatment plan as determined by the interdisciplinary healthcare team.

There are a number of causes of nonadherence among individuals as it relates to their physical or mental care, including:

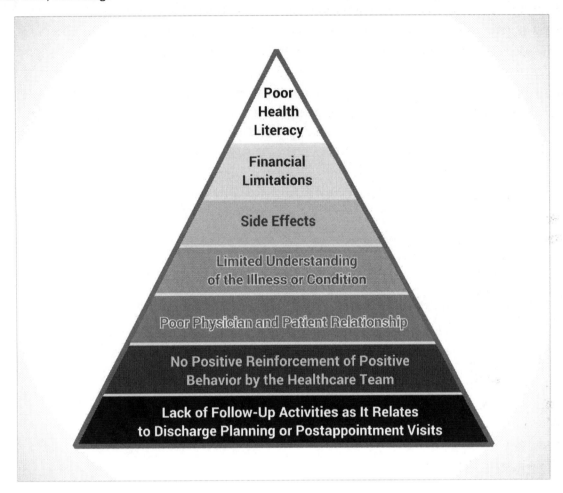

Studies have shown that up to 50% of treatment plan failures are related to a patient's inability to adhere to the prescribed treatment. These poor outcomes are known to contribute to rising healthcare costs, and more than 125,000 deaths are related to medication nonadherence each year.

A **case manager** must understand the influence they have and constantly assess the patient's consistency in adhering to the care regimen and any ongoing barriers he/she might encounter along the way. In order to improve the likelihood of adherence, case managers must possess a unique set of skills, with communication at the top of the list. He/she has to be able to ask the patient the right questions and listen for critical cues that indicate if a goal is being met or if a barrier is creating a risk for nonadherence.

Next, case managers must establish a comprehensive approach, connecting the dots between interventions, adherence, and outcomes. In addition, he/she has to function as an educator who is capable of informing and/or reinforcing the purpose of the treatment plan that has been agreed upon by the patient and the treating provider.

Finally, a case manager must get to know the patient and quickly learn to identify the patient's readiness and ability to adhere to a treatment plan.

Differences in and Application of Age Specific Care

Working with patients of various ages requires specific considerations. For example, pediatric cancer in a child will be treated differently than that same cancer in an adult. While many adults may receive chemotherapy in outpatient settings, children may have to be admitted for that same type of care.

When working with children, the case manager must also include the child's caregivers. Case managers may find themselves focusing on the needs of the patient's caregiver so that the caregiver can give adequate support to their child. When interviewing young children, parental consent is needed, but when possible and age appropriate, children should be actively involved in their own healthcare. Case managers should be aware of state laws concerning age of consent and sharing of information between the adolescent and parent. With children, issues such as divorce and custody agreements should be considered in care plans.

Life Span Considerations

When caring for elderly patients, case managers should provide them with as much autonomy as is safe and appropriate. Elderly patients may also be educated about making advance directives or about selecting a surrogate decision maker if they are declining. As patients get older, many prefer to age in place, and case management for geriatic patients entails considerations to make the patient's home safe and to meet common needs. Case managers for geriatric patients may need to evaluate patient's in-home needs, identify social programs for a patient, and help coordinate services and transportation to appointments..

Alternative Care Facilities

Case managers may provide their services in a variety of settings. Acute care, ambulatory care, home health, long-term care, and wellness programs are just a few examples of settings that a patient may experience along the continuum of care. Involvement in this integrated system of care is a life-long journey for most patients in which they move through a rather extensive and comprehensive array of services related to physical, behavioral, and mental health.

Continuing Care Retirement Communities

Continuing Care Retirement Communities (CCRC) provide the aging population with a plethora of services, from independent-living facilities to assisted-living facilities to skilled-nursing facilities—often all on the same campus. This structure allows residents to transition between facilities or move to a different tier as their health declines.

There are three financial models commonly made available to residents.

- **All-Inclusive Model**: Residents receive both long-term care services and healthcare services.
- **Fee-for-Service Model**: The level of care received is based on the payment for care.

- **Modified Coverage Model**: Residents qualify for long-term care based on a predetermined maximum amount.

Assisted-Living Facilities

Assisted-Living Facilities (ALFs) are a form of long-term care that is available to seniors, also known as an alternative level of care. ALFs enable seniors to remain independent, providing services only as they are needed. It is a level of care that bridges the gap between residing in one's own home and living in a nursing facility. They are favorable because they are less expensive than nursing homes.

In some states, room, board, and amenities (e.g., housekeeping, laundry, transportation) may be covered by the Medicaid Waiver program. For most individuals, these amenities are not covered, funded, or regulated by Medicare or Medicaid. ALFs are predominantly operated by for-profit companies. The cost to reside in an assisted-living facility is related to the amount of care needed by the individual. In 2015, the median annual cost to rent a one-bedroom apartment in an assisted-living facility was estimated at $43,200.

Case managers may serve as a liaison between the facility staff, the patient, and the family throughout the patient's residency, whether it is a short-term or long-term stay.

Not only are ALFs used as a permanent solution for aging adults as their functional dependence increases, but they also serve as a resource for temporary respite care. This can be beneficial for caregivers who still have full-time jobs or are planning to take a vacation.

Types of Assisted-Living Facilities

Group Homes

Group homes come in the form of single-room residences, board and care homes, apartments, or even domiciliary care. These for-profit businesses are available for children (nineteen years or younger) or adults. In some instances, group homes are licensed by states, offering individuals an alternative living environment. Group homes may also be set up for a variety of purposes, such as to care for people with disabilities, those who suffer from chronic mental illness, or elderly dementia patients.

Staffing varies depending on the type of group home. While some homes are staffed twenty-four hours a day, others may have "house parents" on the premises who take on a parenting role.

Adult Foster Care

Adult foster care offers support for the activities of daily living and provides room and board. Managed by sponsoring families or paid caregivers living onsite, adult foster care gives aging residents the opportunity to live in an environment that mimics a home-based setting. In some states, adult foster care may be used as an alternative to long-term care or institutionalized living.

Residential Treatment Facilities

Residential treatment facilities provide access to fully integrated, long-term, intensive treatment for individuals suffering from mental illness, substance abuse, or other behavioral-health issues. This structured environment not only gives patients access to qualified staff but also to peers who can help effectively support ongoing treatment.

Individuals who require such assistance may reside in a residential treatment facility for up to a year. Residential treatment facilities provide participants with access to services that are more intensive than is commonly provided in an outpatient setting.

In a residential setting, the case manager serves as an advocate when the patient is unable to advocate for themselves. The case manager supports activities such as care coordination between various members of the interdisciplinary team and activities associated with discharge planning, so that the patient is able to make a safe transition back into the community and into outpatient services. Even after discharge, the case manager will need to maintain ongoing contact with the member and/or family.

Case Management Models, Process, and Tools

The **case-management process** is a collaborative interaction between case manager and patient. According to CCMC, the case-management process consists of a wide range of activities that include:

- Assessment
- Planning
- Implementation
- Coordination
- Monitoring
- Evaluation
- Outcomes

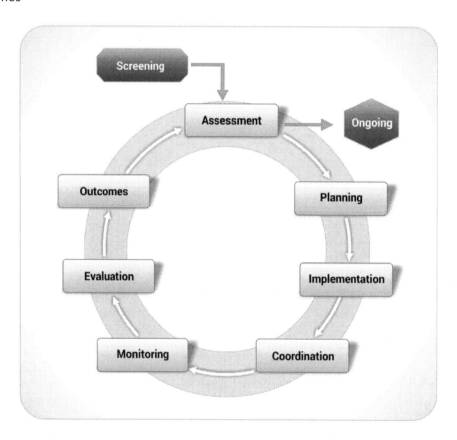

Assessments

The first action a case manager takes during the case-management process is to obtain information about the patient. This is also known as the **assessment**. The assessment process includes gathering information from charts, patients, caregivers, providers, and other members of the healthcare-delivery team where applicable. Health-risk assessments are commonly used to identify the physical and

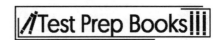

psychosocial health status of the patient. This includes assessing the patient's health-literacy status and deficits as well. The assessment tool used to gather information can vary from organization to organization, though they have similar content. Assessments can provide case managers with a complete view of the patient's current state, along with potential issues and risk factors. They allow case managers to gather relevant information about not only the patient's health and/or psychosocial status but also historical insight into the patient's financial and familial history.

In complex cases, a home assessment may be warranted to ensure that the home environment is stable and safe.

Assessments are not a one-time event. They may be repeated more than once to establish and/or monitor ongoing needs throughout the case-management process. Assessments form the foundation for activities associated with planning, implementation, care coordination, evaluation, and outcomes management.

Planning

During the **planning** process, case managers work in a collaborative fashion with the patient, family, or caregiver, and members of the healthcare-delivery team to develop a plan of care that is cost-effective for the payer or healthcare-delivery system and promotes access to quality care with the best possible outcomes.

As a component of the plan of care, short- and long-term goals are created alongside the patient. These goals must be specific, realistic, and measurable. The patient collaborates with the case manager to prioritize these goals so that they are specific to his/her needs. Goals may be modified during the case-management process due to barriers or complications that arise, but they should remain individualized and specific to the patient and monitored closely, with a secondary or alternative plan in place. For each goal, interventions are identified to support its achievement.

Implementation

Once the plan of care has been created and approved by the patient, payer, treating physician, and any others indicated, **implementation** of that care plan takes place. During the implementation phase of the case-management process, the interventions are facilitated to support the achievement of those goals that were established during the planning process. Examples of interventions carried out by the case manager might include education, daily or weekly follow-ups with the patient, treating provider or caregiver, or care-coordination activities such as referrals or authorization of services. It is during the implementation phase that case managers document the progress of their client and any barriers they are encountering that may cause nonadherence.

Care Coordination

The **care-coordination** phase of the case-management process involves a coordination of activities and services that support the execution of the overall case-management plan. The case manager becomes the nucleus of activity, working with or on behalf of the member, promoting communication, putting services into place, and removing duplicate services or inefficiencies that may impede progress. Case managers provide the patient not only with a connection to the healthcare system but also to community resources.

Monitoring

Case managers must **monitor** the progress of the plan of care and anticipate when modifications may be required to ensure overall effectiveness and the achievement of expected outcomes. Monitoring may also require the case manager to revisit certain phases of the case-management process, such as assessment. In this case, the case manager will need to conduct a reassessment of the patient's overall health or home environment and reprioritize goals in the order of those most critical to the patient or caregiver.

Reassessments might be initiated for a variety of reasons, including changes in the patient's medical or psychosocial status or a need for changed goals.

Evaluation

During the **evaluation** phase of the case-management process, case managers should review the plan of care to determine if the goals and desired outcomes have been achieved. Evaluation is not a one-time event; it should be repetitive and continuous, with the case manager not only looking to determine if goals are being achieved but also evaluating the patient's quality of life. Other things to be evaluated are cost savings, overall effectiveness, and outcomes associated with case-management activities.

Documentation during the evaluation and case-management process should always be objective when identifying whether or not goals were met.

Outcomes

Outcome tracking is an essential activity of case management. The value of case management is documented by the measurement of outcomes, requiring case managers to collect various forms of outcome data. This may include information such as patient satisfaction, core measures, HEDIS measures, return to work, quality of care, utilization of services, cost, cost savings, and clinical information. Outcomes information allows organizations, departments, and case managers to make decisions about the validity of programs and the best practices that can ultimately impact the population's health.

Case managers can use outcome data to demonstrate the relationship between case-management interventions to the overall results achieved. Ideally, case managers will have documented a baseline assessment of the patient's condition at the time he/she entered case management, so that any improvement is apparent when the case manager or organization begins a look-back period of the progress of the case. Results achieved should demonstrate an improvement in health status, as well as self-care abilities for a complex patient with multiple comorbidities and changes in the functional status of individuals with behavioral-health conditions.

Case Closure

Once it has been determined that the patient has achieved his/her best level of function, the case manager will make the decision to close the case. Additional factors that must be considered for **case closure** include but are not limited to:

- Risk for readmission
- Services in place or sufficiently delivered to meet the needs of the patient
- The patient's ability to adequately administer self-care
- The patient's ability to adhere to care
- The patient's support system
- The patient's action plan in place for an urgent or emergent event
- The patient's demonstrated understanding of how to seek healthcare support through the appropriate channels

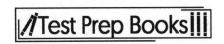

On occasion, case managers may close cases in which the following occurs:

- The patient dies.
- Benefits or eligibility for services are terminated.
- The patient or caregiver declines case-management services.
- Services are no longer available.

Coding Methodologies

Diagnosis-Related Groups

Diagnosis-Related Groups (DRGs) are used to categorize patients based on their diagnoses, types of treatment—including surgical procedures—and the presence or absence of comorbidities or complications. Clinicians and organizations such as hospitals and managed care organizations use DRGs to help with determining what constitutes an acceptable duration or length of stay based on their diagnosis. Hospital stays are also assigned a DRG. Diagnosis-related groups additionally relate the case mix (the variety of cases handled) of a healthcare organization to the expense of providing medical care and are used to help healthcare providers receive appropriate financial reimbursement from health insurance organizations like Medicare. A patient's DRG is determined using ICD-10 diagnostic codes.

Diagnostic and Statistical Manual of Mental Disorders (DSM)

The **Diagnostic and Statistical Manual of Mental Disorders** (DSM-5) functions as the standard system of classification of mental disorders. Comprising three major components—the diagnostic classification, the diagnostic criteria sets, and the descriptive text—the DSM is used by mental-health professionals and other healthcare professionals, including case managers, to classify mental illness. The DSM contains diagnoses that include a diagnostic code typically used by individual providers, institutions, and agencies for data-collection and billing purposes.

International Classification of Diseases (ICD)

Under the **International Classification of Diseases** (ICD), Tenth Revision, or ICD-10, codes are assigned to help classify individuals into manageable categories that have clinical meaning. The ICD-10 is a standard diagnostic tool that is leveraged to track epidemiology, support health management, and guide clinical activities. Healthcare professionals and organizations alike find the ICD-10 tool to be beneficial as it allows for the ability to closely track both the incidence and prevalence of diseases, along with other health problems that may impact various populations.

The ICD-10 is used in more than a hundred countries and operates as a means for identifying health trends and statistics all over the world, and it allows for countries to compare and exchange health information using a common language.

ICD-10, implemented in 2015, allows providers to gain a deeper level of detail about a patient's condition. The ICD is updated periodically to reflect advances in health and medical science. The ICD-11 will be finalized and/or released in 2018.

Current Procedural Terminology

Current Procedure Terminology, commonly referred to as CPT, is a medical code that is utilized along with ICD numerical diagnostic coding as a component of the billing process. CPT codes are used to identify medical, surgical, and diagnostic procedures and services for entities such as physicians, health-insurance companies, and accreditation organizations.

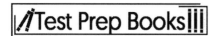

Continuum of Care/Continuum of Health and Human Services/Social Services

The **continuum of care** (CoC) requires integrated case management for patients in multiple settings, over a period of time. It happens from birth to the start of an illness to the point in which the patient is either no longer ill or the patient is no longer eligible for medical or case-management services.

The continuum of care encompasses a wide range of services, including acute care, ambulatory care, home care, extended care, and wellness programs. The CoC supports the goal of providing integrated health services that are cost-effective for complex patients with chronic conditions, providing them with greater access to services.

Given the multiple settings in which a patient may reside, case managers may be required to communicate with other case managers in meeting physical or psychosocial needs.

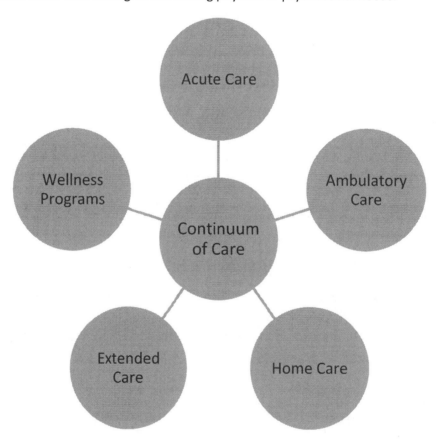

In case management, patients are at greatest risk during the transition between points of care; specifically, when they are transitioning from one level of care to another. Case managers play a critical role in ensuring that these transitions are as seamless as possible. This is only achievable with effective discharge planning or, in some instances, end-of-life planning. Case managers must anticipate the needs of a patient as he/she moves between various levels of care.

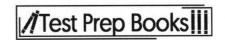

Case Managers as Advocates

Throughout the continuum of care, case managers must function as advocates and place the needs of the patient ahead of their own beliefs or, in some instances, that of the organization for which they work. This can put case managers in a precarious position in which they are working against their company's vision for the good of the patient.

Case Managers as Educators

Case managers also spend a great deal of time educating patients and families, not only about the complexity of a patient's condition but also about the various services for which they are eligible.

Patient and Family Empowerment

Throughout the CoC, case managers will find that they must also empower patients and/or caregivers so they eventually attain independence by demonstrating decision-making and self-care skills.

Case Managers as Communicators and Collaborators

Case managers must demonstrate good written and verbal skills throughout the CoC. Case managers are often the liaison between the patient and the provider, thus making effective communication a necessity. While a good case manager knows when and how to be assertive, he/she must be careful not to appear too aggressive. Instead, he or she serves as an ambassador of good will who has the best interests of both the patient and provider at heart.

Case managers are also required to function as collaborators. Although this can prove to be a time-consuming task, the long-term benefits of establishing trust with various stakeholders are well worth the energy.

Cost-Containment Principles

Case managers have a role in cost containment, which essentially means keeping treatment costs to a minimum. While they act as advocates to get the best treatment for their patients, case managers must also find the treatment option that is most financially feasible for the patient and, in some instances, the insurance organization. Case management can support efforts to reduce costs and reduce spending, moving toward the ultimate goal of cost containment and/or reduction. When deployed in the right manner, case-management activities can:

- Identify barriers to care.
- Prevent hospital readmissions.
- Support care optimization.
- Stabilize patients.

Cost savings are not always obvious or easy to document. Any cost savings that are documented must be accurate and defensible when presenting the effectiveness of case management.

Cost containment is an effort to ensure that the medical coverage provided through insurance is as comprehensive yet inexpensive as possible. Depending on the goal of cost containment, sometimes the result is a greater cost for the patient and sometimes for the insurance company, medical provider, or employer. Some cost containment strategies are used by insurance companies, such as **co-pays**, which are the fixed fees patients have to pay for different services, like a doctor's visit. Another strategy insurance companies use for cost containment is **deductibles**, or the minimum amount that must be paid by the patient before the insurance kicks in. **Co-insurance** is another important aspect of cost containment and refers to the percentage of treatment costs paid by the insurance company and the percentage that has to be paid by the patient. While organizations and insurance companies are attempting to keep their own costs to a minimum by placing more of the cost burden on the patient, the case manager should work to find the option that will best achieve cost containment for the patient.

Healthcare providers usually have agreements with specific insurance companies and utilize different types of insurance, which must be considered when the patient is seeking treatment. **Preferred provider organizations** (PPOs) are those medical providers that have contracts with specific insurance companies. As a result, these providers usually have better rates and lower costs for the patient when it comes to co-pays and deductibles. Similarly, **health maintenance organizations** (HMOs) function on a prepaid basis, covering a fixed amount for treatment for the year. HMOs seek the lowest costs by approving only those treatments they deem necessary and by encouraging preventative care. Medicare and Medicaid, along with other health plans, reimburse hospitals depending on a patient's Diagnosis-Related Group (DRG). This provides incentive for the hospital to keep costs lower. Navigating the system and understanding which insurance and treatment options are most cost-effective can often be a significant challenge for the patient. Case managers should assist with this process and help their patients obtain the best possible insurance option and find appropriate service providers within their coverage area.

Factors Used to Identify Client's Acuity or Severity Levels

Case-managed patients are generally assigned an **acuity level rating** that indicates the severity of an illness or disability. Acuity levels assist case managers in identifying how sick a patient is at the time of case-management engagement. Acuity levels are generally assigned using a set of criteria that has been established by the organization for which they work. Data gained during the initial intake screening coupled with the level of services required by the patients over a short-term period can aid in establishing the assigned acuity level for a patient.

Currently, there is no standing acuity model or program that is utilized by all healthcare-delivery systems, but rather there are various models, software, tools, and resources used by various agencies to determine acuity. They do share a common core of criteria, however, that may be utilized to define the acuity of a case-management patient.

Acuity levels can assist both case managers and departments in monitoring a case manager's caseload and ensuring the case manager maintains a proper caseload mix. Ultimately, there should be an equal distribution of cases per acuity level.

In addition, acuity levels can inform decisions made regarding the case-management model used by an organization, as well as the staffing levels maintained to support their programs.

Acuity measures can be helpful in predictive modeling within an organization, such as a managed care organization. Predictive modeling analyzes data received from health-insurance claims, service authorizations, pharmacy utilization, and health-risk assessments to identify the potential risk an individual might have for over utilization of services or facing a catastrophic event.

Most predictive-modeling programs generate risk scores that enable case managers and organizations to prioritize patients and identify the level of care required to achieve stabilization.

Financial Resources

The **financial resources** used to pay for healthcare expenses may vary to include waiver programs, special needs trusts, and viatical settlements.

Waiver Programs

Many states offer Medicaid Waiver Programs, which allow for the provision of long-term care services in the home and community. **Waiver programs** are a combination of standard medical and nonmedical services. Examples of the services provided by waiver programs include case management, home health aide, personal-attendant care services, adult day health services, respite care, and residential care. On occasion, states may choose to include additional value-added services.

Special Needs Trusts

Special-needs trusts (SNTs) are managed by one individual on behalf of someone else. Specifically, they are designed to benefit the disabled or mentally ill. SNTs are designed to support those who lack the mental capacity to manage his/her own finances. They can greatly assist with preventing loss of government benefits. Trustees of special needs trusts may be family members or third parties who are appointed by the court.

Special-needs trusts can benefit the recipient because they keep disabled individuals from being disqualified from receiving Supplemental Security Income (SSI), Medicaid, vocational rehabilitation, and subsidized housing. A special-needs trust protects the individual from being disqualified.

A trustee may seek support from a case manager so that he/she can provide an initial and annual assessment. The case manager may be asked to function as a liaison between the patient/family and the provider or to help educate the trustee about those services or programs available to the patient.

Viatical Settlements

Viatical settlements take place when an individual elects to sell his/her life-insurance policy for more than the cash surrender value, in order to immediately obtain cash. Viatical settlements are available in all fifty states and may be sold by individuals facing a terminal illness to relieve their financial burdens. There are viatical companies that will offer to buy policies directly while others may purchase the policy from another funding source. For example, someone with less than six months to live might be offered 80% of the policy's face value. Case managers can assist their clients in obtaining accurate information related to viatical settlements.

Goals and Objectives of Case-Management Practice

Case management has a set of goals at the core of its practice, and they are as follows:

- Support and facilitate improved access to care.
- Provide service and care coordination.
- Promote care that is medically necessary and cost-effective.
- Create a pathway to functional stability.
- Empower the client to engage in self-directed care.

Case managers should diligently work to assess high-risk conditions and behavior, partner with the patient or caregiver to formulate a collaborative and effective treatment plan, and monitor for outcomes. The goal for case managers is for clients to achieve and maintain optimal levels of physical and mental health and functioning. This is primarily accomplished as the case manager works on behalf of the client and plays a supportive role in the client's treatment.

Case managers usually serve in a coordination capacity, connecting the client to a variety of services to meet his/her physical, medical, psychological, and social needs. The case manager is responsible for managing the overall plan of treatment and care, which may include involvement with multiple providers, physicians, and community resources. The case manager does not directly provide all the services that a client may need but is responsible for ensuring the client receives quality care and any necessary treatment through the appropriate resources.

Another important objective of case management is the empowerment of the client. Rather than making decisions on his/her behalf, a case manager collaborates with the client on treatment plans and goals and seeks to empower the client in self-directed care. The goal of case management is not to cause the client to become dependent on the case manager, but rather to help the client become independent, fully involved in his/her own treatment process, and able to engage in self-advocacy. This includes providing education for the client around his/her own illness or disability and equipping the client with the information necessary to take charge of his/her care and treatment.

Healthcare Delivery Systems

The United States' **healthcare-delivery system** comprises several subsystems. Access to quality healthcare is strongly driven by health-insurance coverage, location, and technology-driven systems. Legal risks can often influence the behavior of healthcare professionals.

Healthcare-delivery systems in the United States can be categorized in the following way:

Managed Care

Managed care is considered to be the dominant healthcare-delivery system in the United States. Managed care seeks to:

- Control costs by managing utilization of services.
- Regulate provider reimbursement.
- Establish efficiency with integrated healthcare practices.

Managed care organizations (MCOs) are financed by employers or government agencies by way of a contract. Through the contract, MCOs provide a set of healthcare services to members who are enrolled in the health plan. Members, also known as enrollees, are covered by the contracted health plan for a wide spectrum of services.

MCOs negotiate with providers to accept a capitation rate (in most instances) and provide members with a discounted rate. Providers agree to join a network of treating physicians and treat MCO members.

Military

Active-duty military personnel in the United States Army, Navy, Air Force, and Coast Guard, along with other uniformed nonmilitary services, receive medical care that is free of charge. The **military healthcare system** is integrated and provides comprehensive health treatment. In many instances, medical services are provided by individuals who are also in the military or in other uniformed services.

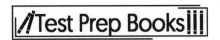

Families and dependents of active-duty or retired career military personnel may also receive care at facilities like hospitals or clinics through TRICARE coverage. **TRICARE** is an insurance plan that enables enrollees, also known as beneficiaries, to receive medical or mental-health treatment in nonmilitary facilities.

The **VA** or **Veterans Administration** healthcare system makes healthcare available to retired veterans with previous military service. Disabled veterans are given priority under this system and have access to hospital care, mental-health services, and long-term care.

Vulnerable Populations

Those who are poor, uninsured, or reside in geographic locations that are economically disadvantaged are identified as being among the most vulnerable population. **Vulnerable populations** receive care from settings that are specially designed to support their needs and include health centers. Additionally, physician's offices, hospitals, outpatient clinics, and emergency departments provide a "safety net" of providers who are equipped to provide comprehensive medical treatment.

Medicare

Medicare serves approximately 39 million people. Those who qualify for Medicare are 65 years of age or older or have been diagnosed with end-stage renal disease or a disability.

Medicare is composed of three parts:

1. Part A. **Medicare Part A** provides coverage to Medicare recipients for healthcare that is received at hospitals, hospice care, or nursing facilities, as well as some home healthcare services. There are no monthly premiums.

2. Part B. **Medicare Part B** provides coverage at an additional monthly premium for physician services and some outpatient services that are not included with Part A.

3. Part D - The **Medicare Prescription Drug Plan**. The Medicare Prescription Drug Plan provides Medicare recipients with coverage for brand-name and generic prescription drugs at participating pharmacies, which helps to reduce the cost of ordinarily high-cost drugs or medications that would otherwise prove burdensome for the recipient.

Medicaid

Medicaid provides health insurance to the disabled, children, the elderly, and low-income men and women. Some Medicaid recipients (older adults and those with disabilities) may qualify for long-term care services.

SCHIP

Established in 1997, the **State Children's Health Insurance Program** (SCHIP) provides coverage for those children whose families do not qualify for Medicaid due to income levels. Services covered include:

- Physician visits
- Hospital stays
- Emergency room visits

There are communities in which the number of available "safety net" providers are limited or not available, which results in a greater risk for vulnerable populations.

<u>Integrated Service Delivery</u>

Integrated delivery systems (IDSs) have become a gold standard in the United States because of their ability to establish and maintain a strong and strategic network of hospitals, physicians, and insurers.

Hospice, Palliative, and End-of-Life Care

End-of-life issues refer to the treatment and care people receive when they have a terminal or chronic illness or are approaching the end of their lives. It is the goal of health professionals and all those providing end-of-life care to ensure that the patient's last days of life are as painless and comfortable as possible. One focus is on physical care, especially pain management and dealing with common symptoms of terminal illness, such as fatigue, constipation, sleep and appetite issues, and nausea. The other aspect is psychosocial care: addressing spiritual or existential concerns, relationship problems, fears about the process of dying, loss of independence, and mental health matters, such as anxiety or depression. Palliative care and hospice care are carried out by collaborative interdisciplinary teams of doctors, nurses, social workers, clinicians, and others.

<u>Hospice Care</u>

Hospice care is typically administered as a component of end-of-life care to those who are suffering from terminal illness with less than six months to live. It is estimated that approximately 1.5 million people receive hospice care in a single year. Individuals who receive hospice care typically have received a diagnosis for a condition that has no cure. A component of hospice care may include palliative care. The goal in providing hospice care is not to provide a cure but to ensure that the patient's remaining days are as comfortable as possible.

Both the patient and the family should be considered clients of a hospice organization. Hospice is available to provide support for both the family and the patient. Families may receive grief counseling.

Studies have shown that some patients improve with hospice services. Recipients of hospice services may stay in their home environment or services may also be provided in a nursing-home setting.

Hospice patients and their families can receive care for six months or longer and, most importantly, they have the option of keeping their treating physician involved with the care that is being provided.

Coverage through Medicare or other insurance providers usually covers the last six months of a person's life. This can hinder access to treatment because a time-specific prognosis is very difficult, so people usually receive care for a shorter time frame than the six months for which they qualify.

<u>Palliative Care</u>

Palliative care is comprehensive care provided for symptoms and illnesses exacerbated by chronic conditions, including cancer, liver failure, dementia, and chronic obstructive pulmonary disease. Palliative care is delivered by a multidisciplinary team of physicians, nurses, nutritionists, pharmacists, social workers, case managers, and a number of specialists in a collaborative manner.

The characteristic that distinguishes palliative care from hospice care is the time at which palliative care may be offered. Case managers may advocate for palliative care to be administered at any stage of an illness or at any age. Ideally, palliative care should be initiated upon diagnosis for conditions like cancer and continue for the duration of therapy, follow-up care, and end-of-life care, as indicated.

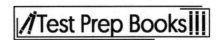

Palliative care has the ability to improve one's quality of life, addressing physical, behavioral, spiritual, and practical needs. Palliative care delivers a variety of options to patients that go far beyond pain assessments.

Palliative care may be delivered in the patient's home as long as they are under the supervision of a physician, or it may be a component of hospice or provided in a long-term facility. It is typically covered by health insurance and in some instances may be covered by Medicare and Medicaid. Those who do not qualify for palliative care by any of the identified entities may need further assistance from their case manager and/or social worker to identify potential resources that can provide the necessary support to receive services.

End-of-Life Care

Patients should be encouraged to discuss **end-of-life** wishes with their family members early on in the process when possible. The decision-making process can be complex, intense, and stressful for those left to make the decision for the patient. Having a plan in place that makes the patient's wishes clear can reduce the level of stress for both the family and the patient.

It is helpful for the patient to establish a plan that outlines specifically what his/her wishes are as relates to end-of-life care. A healthcare proxy can assist with ensuring such wishes are honored. Core topics and/or decisions a healthcare proxy can assist with include the location of healthcare (e.g., at home or in a facility) and resuscitation expectations.

Case managers may need to provide guidance in pointing their patients in the right direction to complete an advanced directive and/or living will. Advanced directives and living wills are two additional resources that should be kept on file to assist with the documentation and communication of a patient's wishes.

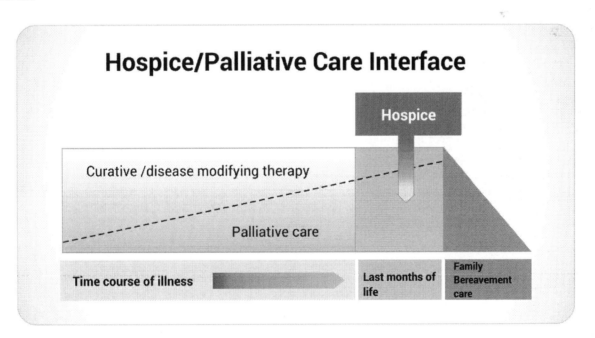

A **Do Not Resuscitate** (DNR) order prevents health workers from administering CPR on an individual whose heart has stopped or who has stopped breathing. A person may choose to have a DNR order if they have a late-stage terminal illness and the attempts to resuscitate could decrease quality of life or be unlikely to succeed. **Withdrawal of care** happens when a decision is made to stop the life-sustaining support that is being provided, such as a ventilator. This decision is often made when life is being artificially sustained but there is no chance of improvement or recovery. These difficult decisions are made by the patient, or by the family, if the patient is incapable of making the decision. When case managers are discussing this issue with patients, it is important to ensure that patients make the decision based on their own values and wishes. While the medical facts should be fully presented to contribute to an informed decision-making process, there should be no coercion or undue influence. Ultimately, it is the decision of the patient, or the family.

Insurance Principles

Insurance can be broken down into four subcategories: health, disability, long-term, and workers' compensation.

Health Insurance

Health insurance provides individuals with access to healthcare in a variety of healthcare settings. Health insurance covers those costs associated with medical and surgical expenses as well as treatments. It may pay a portion or all of those costs. The insured individual may be required to pay for costs out-of-pocket and be later reimbursed. Healthcare insurance can protect the insured from high medical costs.

Most people in the United States receive health insurance through their employer. However, some individuals purchase health insurance on their own or have to seek health coverage through government-funded programs like Medicaid and Medicare. The Affordable Care Act has assisted in extending health insurance to individuals in the United States who otherwise may not have qualified previously.

Disability Insurance

Disability insurance is typically distributed as a form of health insurance when an individual is unable to work due to injury or illness. Disability insurance is available in two forms—short term and long term—and is plan specific. **Short-term disability** (STD) is a set of benefits leveraged to provide coverage for an individual during a time in which they are deemed disabled. Unless otherwise indicated, STD is administered over a period of time to not exceed two years.

Long-term disability (LTD) is generally issued to a group or to an individual. LTD is used to replace income lost as a result of a chronic condition or illness.

Long Term Care

Long-term care insurance is insurance that covers care that is received in a nursing home, home health setting, or assisted living facility due to a chronic health condition. Certain patients may not qualify for long-term care insurance if they have pre-existing conditions. While the ACA prohibits other types of insurance from denying patients due to preexisting conditions, this does not apply to long-term care insurance. Most research advocates for the mid 50s being the best age to buy long-term care insurance, as premiums for long-term care insurance rapidly increase with each year of life. Long-term care insurance is most needed by middle-class Americans, as high-income families can often afford care and low-income families qualify for Medicaid.

Workers' Compensation

Established with the enactment of the Workers' Compensation Act in 1911, **Workers' Compensation** is a state-governed insurance that manages work-related injuries.

With the evolution of managed care and case management has come the evolution of workers' compensation, which now often takes on a medical-management model. The distinction between traditional medical-management case management and that of workers' compensation, however, is directly driven by state laws. Case managers for workers' compensation must abide by state laws. While the statutes associated with workers' compensation may vary from state to state, the general framework associated with the practices of workers' compensation is the same.

In addition, workers' compensation does not carry a deductible or co-pay. Patients are able to see their physician of choice, and there is no limit on medical coverage; these cases can be rife with litigation.

Wage-Loss Benefits Coordination

Employers may play a role in coordinating **wage-loss payments** under workers' compensation with Social Security Disability Income (SSDI) or long-term disability insurance. The carrier is required to educate employees of their benefits under SSDI should it be determined that there is some potential for eligibility.

Role of Case Managers in Workers' Compensation

While many cases do not require case-management intervention, it is important to note that case-management activities should begin upon initial report for those that do.

Ultimately, case managers for workers' compensation should aim to monitor for:

- A demonstrated progression toward returning to work
- Adherence and compliance with the agreed-upon treatment plan
- Avoidance of activities by the client that would prevent them from returning to work

Case managers with a background in medical surgical settings have the ability to function as a strong advocate for both workers' compensation organizations and injured parties. Case managers have a role in improving the communication channels between the multiple stakeholders involved in the case, including the injured worker, specialists, primary-care physicians, the carrier, the employer, and other members of the healthcare-delivery team. If it is determined that an employee is using drugs/alcohol at the time an injury occurs, workers' compensation claims may be denied.

Reinsurance

Reinsurance, also known as stop-loss insurance, is a method used to reduce risk or net liability. It is intended to prevent loss in catastrophic cases that could put an insurance company at risk for losing an amount of money that is so significant it could cause them to go bankrupt. Reinsurance is purchased by insurance companies from designated reinsurance carriers.

For example, a company may set aside $500,000 per covered life and set a limit of $50,000 with the reinsurer insurance company. The health insurer would cover claims of up to $50,000 and anything over the $50,000 limit would be reimbursed by the stop-loss carrier for up to a total dollar amount of $500,000.

Long-Term Care

Long-term care services become necessary when individuals are unable to take care of their functional needs as a direct result of a disabling chronic illness or injury. These activities may include but are not limited to bathing, meal preparation, shopping, getting into a chair, or getting into bed. Individuals with developmental disabilities or mental illnesses may also require long-term care services.

Long-term care insurance covers services that are not usually covered by health insurance. It is administered when clinical deficits are present—such as an inability to complete activities of daily living (ADLs) or cognitive impairment.

While some policies offer long-term care insurance for as long as an individual lives, many policies do have limits in place as it relates to the duration for which they will cover services. For example, some will only provide long-term care services over a period of two to five years. A set of criteria must be met in order to qualify for the services, including a deficiency in the following areas:

- Activities of daily living to a specified degree
- Cognitive impairments including short-term or long-term memory orientation and judgment

Those who do not qualify for long-term care services under the ADL or cognitive-impairment umbrellas may qualify to receive them as a result of a medical-necessity clause in their contract.

Forty-one percent of those who access long-term care services are under the age of sixty-five. Case managers providing services to individuals with access to long-term care services can assist their patients in ensuring that they have and/or maintain the appropriate level of services so that they are able to remain in the community and/or in their homes.

Potential long-term services covered may include:

- Home modifications
- Ramp installations
- Emergency response systems
- Respite care
- Home safety assessments
- Skilled-nursing facilities
- Hospice
- Adult day care
- Transitional living centers

Interdisciplinary/Interprofessional Care Team

The **interdisciplinary care team** (ICT) is a collaborative group of healthcare professionals from different backgrounds, disciplines, and professions with the common goal of establishing an effective plan of care. Patients and families should be integral members of the care team and fully involved in the decision-making process. The ICT may include doctors, nurses, psychologists, social workers, dieticians, and family members. Case managers have a role in this team in that they can provide critical information that may lend itself to the shared-decision-making process in establishing the best treatment plan for a patient.

ICTs are becoming more and more of a necessity for a variety of reasons, including but not limited to the following:

- Aging adults with chronic, complex, comorbid conditions

- The need for a team with varying skill sets, knowledge, and abilities to manage patient populations with complex needs

- New policies and evidence-based best practices for managing chronically-ill and disabled populations

- The trend of increased specialization among healthcare professionals

It is important to reinforce that the ICT is a collaborative group that conducts shared decision making. Power should be distributed among individual team members when formulating a plan of care to meet the needs of the patient. However, the distribution of power may create some challenges in those instances where the client has a set of comorbid conditions in both the medical and behavioral domains. Conflict may arise between different professionals as to the best course of action. Despite the potential challenges, these teams tend to be more effective and comprehensive, as well as more cost-effective over the long term.

Levels of Care and Care Settings

Acute Care

Acute care is accessed in an effort to resolve an immediate and unanticipated health event or complex health issue, avoid death, and prevent disability, while simultaneously improving health and promoting wellness. Acute care services are provided in a hospital setting but may also be delivered in other settings based on the acuity of the patient.

Acute care encompasses the following types of services:

- **Emergency care** consists of medical care provided to those experiencing symptoms, illness, or injuries that require immediate attention and may become life threatening if left untreated.

- **Urgent care** is provided to those with an illness or condition that requires immediate attention but does not equate to the necessity of an emergency care visit.

- **Critical care** is provided to those with an illness or injury that is detrimental to life and requires constant monitoring.

- **Trauma care** and **acute-care** surgery provide emergency operative care for life-threatening health issues that require surgery within twenty-four hours of admission.

- **Short-term stabilization** provides immediate acute-care services to those in distress so that they can be transferred to another level of treatment.

Long-Term Care Services

Long-term care services offer a variety of options to those who require services that are designed to provide ongoing support for complex conditions that impact their ability to care for themselves and function independently.

Long-term care encompasses the following types of services:

- **Residential** facilities provide support and/or custodial care to those who are unable to live independently and may have a mental or physical condition.

- **Nursing homes** provide services for those who do not require hospitalization but are unable to remain in their homes to receive care.

- **Assisted living** provides housing for seniors who require minimal assistance with their activities of daily living such as bathing, dressing and eating.

- **Adult/pediatric day health services** provide social engagement for participants as well as caregiver respite services.

- **Subacute care facilities** and **skilled nursing** provide complex care to patients who are medically stable but no longer require acute hospital care, providing them with additional time to improve their ability to function independently and safely prior to being discharged to home. Examples of the type of care provided in this setting include wound care, intravenous therapy, and rehabilitation services.

- **Long-term acute care (LTAC)** provides care to patients following an inpatient acute-care stay with an average length of stay ranging from twenty-five to thirty days.

- **Hospice care** provides end-of-life care to those who have been given a prognosis of six months or less.

It is critical that effective assessments are conducted and ongoing evaluation done so that patients are always provided with the level of care that they need. Discharge and transitional planning at each stage must also be done thoroughly to ensure a patient is adequately prepared for a less intense level of care.

Managed Care Concepts

About Managed Care Organizations (MCOs)

The role of **managed care organizations** (MCOs) is to manage the financing and delivery of medically necessary health services. MCOs connect patients to providers that can give them the treatment they need.

Their responsibilities include:

- Facilitation of healthcare delivery to health-plan members
- Appropriate reimbursement for services delivered
- Ensuring members have access to appropriate services

MCOs promote cost control and are designed to make healthcare more affordable and accessible. The result is lower out-of-pocket expenses and lower premiums. Payers determine which providers their members may access by establishing a network.

Members are encouraged to see primary-care physicians for their routine care and to only seek specialists under the referral of their primary-care physician. Urgent care centers are the preferred place of treatment for urgent care needs, as opposed to visits to the emergency room.

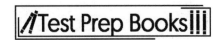

Managed care organizations utilize case-management services to ensure that members of the MCO are receiving the right services, in the right location, at the right time. MCOs take it a step further to ensure that those services are medically necessary by using industry-recognized national criteria like InterQual and Milliman. These criteria sets enable organizations to determine if a member's illness or condition warrants the level of service being received. Again, the ultimate goal is to not only ensure the member is receiving the appropriate level of care but to also keep costs down.

MCO Case Managers

MCO case managers play a vital role in their organization. They oversee the care that members receive and closely monitor the dollars spent. Case managers collaborate with others within the organization to arrange for authorization of services and validate whether or not the treatment plans in place are adequate.

MCOs may carry out services in a variety of ways. Many MCOs provide case management that is targeted in nature, focusing on those populations that pose the greatest risk due to complexity or risk for catastrophic outcomes. Case managers within the MCO have the unique responsibility of balancing the needs of the payer, physician, and patient to achieve the best possible results. Case managers operate as generalists, but some MCOs elect to use specialist case managers when possible.

NCQA, the **National Commission for Quality Assurance**, influences MCO strategies and the methods by which these organizations facilitate case-management services. NCQA challenges MCOs to implement programs such as disease-management programs that demonstrate a real improvement in health status, using industry-recognized guidelines and best practices.

The evaluation of an MCO program can be done using a variety of tools, including internal audits, documentation of best practices that demonstrate positive trends within the populations that are being managed, and those activities that lead to a reduction in inpatient bed days, admissions, and ER visits.

Health Maintenance Organization (HMO)

Health maintenance organizations (HMOs) provide access to healthcare services in a select region to individuals enrolled in a health plan. HMOs collect payments for each of their members and provide access to standard inpatient and ambulatory care services.

Some HMOs have open-access models in which members are allowed to access any provider in the network without needing to seek care from their PCP, either using a self-referral or the standard PCP referral. Other HMOs have open panels in which physicians obtain and maintain contracts through Independent Practice Associations. In the staff model, HMOs hire physicians themselves, and providers are only allowed to care for members within the health plan. Finally, some HMOs follow a group model, sometimes referred to as a closed model. In this case, the HMO has a contract with a group of doctors. These doctors can then divide profits.

Independent Practice Association (IPA)

IPAs or **Independent Practice Associations** consist of a group of physicians who are organized to support HMOs and provide services to those enrolled. IPAs are favorable for doctors because they provide a degree of independence. Despite having an exclusive contract in place with the HMO, IPAs can see patients who are not enrolled with the HMO, therefore giving them access to patients from a variety of sources and settings, and from multiple contract agreements. Under the IPA model, HMOs can establish a relationship with all the physicians in the group even if there is a single contract in place. IPAs receive reimbursement through a capitated payment or fee-for-services model.

Preferred Provider Organization (PPO)

Preferred provider organizations or PPOs are more flexible than the HMO model. PPOs permit out-of-network provider visits and patients can obtain a degree of coverage for these visits. The PPO referral process is also a bit easier because it does not require referral to see a specialist nor is there a requirement to choose a primary-care physician.

Point of Service Plans (POS)

A **point of service** plan is a fusion of the best characteristics of the HMO and PPO plans in managed care. While participants have an in-network provider who functions as their primary-care provider (PCP), they can access care outside of their network with a referral from the PCP, at a cost.

POS plans may be upwards of fifty percent cheaper than PPOs. However, they are not able to provide the same robust network of healthcare providers as commonly seen with a PPO or HMO. Deductibles can be expensive with this model, and the administrative burden is incredibly frustrating to those who dare to venture out of network. This leads to longer wait times for reimbursement, increased delays associated with some referrals, and a higher rate of co-pays.

Management of Clients with Acute and Chronic Illness(es)

It is not uncommon for individuals to have more than one chronic illness. These are sometimes referred to as **comorbid conditions** because they exist at the same time and may or may not have a direct relationship with one another. For example, someone who is a "brittle diabetic," currently struggling to manage his/her health condition may also have other diagnoses that are occurring at the same time, including depression or cardiovascular disease. Case managers who are providing services to clients with multiple chronic illnesses must be consistent in their application of the case-management process. Chronic conditions tend to go through cycles of stability and exacerbation, in some instances with irreversible disease progression.

Case managers who provide services to the chronically ill and disabled require an increased level of awareness, education, and support because these conditions significantly impact the client's overall and long-term well-being, especially among those who are suffering from multiple chronic illnesses. Chronic illnesses may stabilize but may not necessarily be resolved. For example, someone who has a diagnosis of diabetes may very well stabilize and control blood sugar, but his/her condition always has the potential to become unstable if not managed appropriately. In the case of multiple chronic conditions, all the challenges and complications of long-term illness are exacerbated. The patient will have even more difficulty managing the social, emotional, vocational, and physical domains of life.

Case managers must be aware, educated and able to provide meaningful support in these ways:

- Identify the complications associated with different chronic conditions.
- Demonstrate an awareness of proper diagnostic testing and procedures.
- Demonstrate an understanding of current treatment options for all diagnoses.
- Verbalize an awareness of expected outcomes.
- Encourage client self-management, empowerment, and self-directed care.

Case managers may be required to play a role in helping clients understand their conditions and the potential impact those conditions have on the client's physical, behavioral, and social well-being. Case managers will also need to be prepared to assist in empowering patients to work towards self-management. A client with multiple conditions will have even more providers involved in their care, so it is imperative that the client is able to engage in self-advocacy and treatment coordination. **Self-management** is when the client takes an active role in care-coordination activities, which can ultimately reduce the risk of disorganized healthcare experiences and unnecessary healthcare costs.

Self-management can only be effective, however, if healthcare providers understand what self-management entails and demonstrate consistent support of the patient's efforts to take control of his/her physical and behavioral health. Case managers can influence the success of self-management activities by bridging gaps between the patient, providers, and managed care organizations facilitating the patient's benefits package.

Finally, it is important to recognize the unique struggle for those with multiple chronic illnesses. The risk of mental illness is greater, as they battle feelings of isolation, loneliness, fatigue and hopelessness. Having multiple conditions means more doctors' visits to attend, more medications to manage, and more treatment options to consider. All of these things can be overwhelming to someone who is already struggling with the daily symptoms of illness. The job of case managers is to make sure the client has adequate social and emotional support, including support groups, therapists, and family support.

Management of Clients with Disability(ies)

The main difference between acute and chronic illnesses is duration; acute illnesses are short term and chronic illnesses are long term. **Acute illness** or disability has specific symptoms or areas of focus and can often be treated and recovered from within a limited period of time, if survived. Chronic illnesses, on the other hand, may have less definable and more varied symptoms. It is not easily treated or cured. Those with chronic illnesses or disabilities will need more comprehensive and longer-term care, often throughout the course of their lives. Typically, a chronic illness has a more gradual onset, whereas acute illness is a more sudden onset; however, a chronic illness may come as the result of an acute illness.

In managing patients with an acute illness or disability, the focus is on the cure and on treating the specific symptoms. Along with supporting the patient throughout the process of treatment, the case manager should focus on what happens after treatment or hospitalization. This includes any follow-up physical therapy or rehabilitation that needs to be arranged, as well as living arrangements, short-term living adjustments, etc. Generally, once the disease has been treated, and the patient has successfully readjusted to normal life, little follow up will be needed and the case manager's job may be done.

For those dealing with chronic illness or disability, the case manager will have a different role. In this situation, more emphasis needs to be placed on finding long-term providers and resources for the patient, including nursing care, if necessary. Chronic illness does not just entail short-term adjustments but requires a lifestyle change that accommodates the limitations of the illness. Chronic illness impacts every area of a person's life, including his/her living environment, ability to work, sense of identity, social support system, and level of everyday functioning. The case manager's job is to encourage patient empowerment and self-directed care so that the patient will be able to maintain the best level of health and well-being that is possible. The adjustment to living with a chronic illness can also impact a person's mental health and lead to depression or anxiety.

Case managers should focus on holistic care for the patient, making sure his/her physical, social, and emotional needs are all being met. It is also critical to ensure that the family and caregivers are receiving adequate support, so that they are better able to take care of the patient. In order to make sure the patient has a comprehensive network of resources and support, the case manager must emphasize coordination and effective communication between the patient, family, and all service providers.

Advancements in healthcare have improved the ability to manage and treat acute illnesses and conditions in a timely and cost-effective way that is least devastating to the patient. This has enabled the system to focus more on how to best deliver case management to the chronically ill and disabled.

Medication Safety Assessment, Reconciliation, and Management

Proper medication-therapy management (MTM) and medication reconciliation helps to reduce the risk of medication errors inside and outside of the hospital, facility, or home settings. Patients with chronic conditions, or even those who develop acute conditions, are regularly prescribed new medications. Whether these new medications are based on the need to increase the dosage to alleviate symptoms or to provide relief for new ones, there is a risk of duplicating medications or inadvertently prescribing incorrect dosages.

Medication-therapy management has to do with the patient obtaining and properly taking the medications that are needed. There are various reasons why this does not occur, such as inadequate treatment, lack of finances, or neglecting to take medications that have been prescribed. The case manager's job is to identify any barriers that may exist in the patient's medication-therapy management and help the client to overcome them. **Medication Therapy Management Programs** (MTMP) were established with the US Medicare Modernization Act of 2003 for the primary purpose of promoting medication adherence among Medicare Part D beneficiaries through the use of education and counseling. MTMPs are designed to support those taking medications for chronic conditions. In addition, patients have access to self-management education and two-way communication with the MTM service provider.

Medication reconciliation is the process of documenting the patient's medication regimen, including the name of the medication, dosage, frequency, and route, and then comparing it with the prescribed medication regimen received during the transition of care (i.e., discharge, admission, or transfer). Medication reconciliation provides the opportunity to identify discrepancies and inconsistencies between what the caregiver and/or patient understands to be their treatment regimen and what the healthcare provider has documented as the treatment regimen. Medication reconciliation can identify gaps in the understanding of prescription changes and actual medication-therapy management.

Military and Veteran Benefit Programs

TRICARE

TRICARE is a healthcare management program that operates under the Department of Defense (DoD) and provides coverage to millions of beneficiaries, including active-duty service members of the following:

- Army
- Navy
- Air Force
- Marine Corp
- US Coast Guard
- National Guard/Reserve Members
- National Oceanic and Atmospheric Administration

- Public Health Service
- Survivors
- Former spouses
- Medal of Honor recipients and their families

This program was previously known as CHAMPUS and only provided for eligible persons in limited categories. TRICARE offers a variety of health plans based on the region in which the beneficiary resides and their eligibility, and it exceeds the requirements of the Affordable Care Act.

TRICARE Prime

TRICARE Prime is available to active-duty uniformed service members and their families, activated National Guard and Reserve members, families that become eligible under the Transitional Assistance Management Program, survivors, Medal of Honor recipients and their families, and qualified former spouses. Retired service members and their families may also qualify for TRICARE Prime, unless they are eligible for TRICARE for Life.

Under TRICARE Prime, recipients are assigned a primary-care manager (PCM) who is a network or military provider that provides most of the beneficiaries' care. He/she is responsible for coordinating referrals, accepting copayments, and filing claims on the recipient's behalf.

While active-duty service members do not pay anything out-of-pocket, and active-duty family members only pay if they use a point-of-service option, all other beneficiaries are required to pay annual enrollment fees and network copayments.

ECHO

The **Extended Care Health Option** (ECHO) provides active-duty family members who have a qualifying mental or physical disability with financial assistance. Services provided under this program may include but are not limited to:

- Special education
- Sixteen hours per month of ECHO Respite Care with other authorized ECHO benefits
- Up to forty hours per week of ECHO Respite Care if the family member is homebound
- Durable medical equipment
- Assistive services including interpreter or translation services
- Transportation

Children continue to qualify for ECHO benefits beyond the age of twenty-one or twenty-three as long as a parent remains on active duty or is unable to provide support due to their mental or physical disability.

TRICARE Standard and Extra

Beneficiaries who are enrolled in the Defense Enrollment Eligibility Reporting System (DEERS) are automatically enrolled in **TRICARE Standard**, if eligible. Activated National Guard and Reserve members and their families who become eligible under the Transitional Assistance Management Program, survivors, Medal of Honor recipients and their families, and qualified former spouses are eligible to participate in this program.

TRICARE Reserve Select

TRICARE Reserve Select is a premium-based plan. It is accessible all over the world for Selected Reserve members and their families. Beneficiaries of this program can visit any TRICARE-authorized provider.

They do not require a referral to receive care, but some services may require authorization for services from a regional contractor. Members of the Individual Ready Reserve (IRR) do not qualify for TRICARE Reserve Select.

This plan does require beneficiaries to pay monthly premiums, annual deductibles, or a percentage for those services with coverage.

TRICARE Retired Reserve

TRICARE Retired Reserve is another premium-based plan that is available all over the world for those retired Reserve members who, along with their families or survivors, qualify. Much like TRICARE Reserve Select, this health plan does not require qualifying beneficiaries to obtain a referral for care. However, they may still be required to obtain authorization for services from their regional contractor.

TRICARE for Life

The Department of Defense (DoD) changed the TRICARE program in 2001, granting coverage to those military beneficiaries who were also eligible for Medicare and those who had purchased Medicare Part B. This program became known as the **TRICARE for Life** (TFL) program, functioning as a secondary payer to Medicare.

TRICARE-eligible beneficiaries who receive Medicare Part A and Part B are eligible to receive TFL as a Medicare-wraparound coverage. TRICARE is secondary payer after Medicare in the United States and US territories, but TRICARE for Life is the first payer in overseas areas.

TFL participants can visit any provider they choose. However, out-of-pocket expenses may be higher for those who seek care from VA providers or those providers who do not accept Medicare. VA providers are not permitted to bill Medicare.

TRICARE Young Adult

Young, unmarried adults between the ages of twenty-one and twenty-six years of age can continue to participate in TRICARE based on their sponsor's service status. The program is known as the **TRICARE Young Adult** program.

US Family Health Plan

Another option for beneficiaries is the **US Family Health Plan**. Recipients of this program receive care at a designated community-based, not-for-profit health system. The plan also provides prescription-drug coverage. Physicians treating these beneficiaries must be affiliated with at least one of the US Family Health Plan healthcare systems to provide care. Beneficiaries under this plan would not be able to receive care at military hospitals or clinics within the TRICARE network of providers.

VA

The **Veterans' Administration** (VA) provides eligible veterans access to services that closely relate to their military history, disability rating, and classification at the time of discharge. The VA is perhaps the largest healthcare system in the nation.

CHAMPVA

The CHAMPVA Center in Denver, Colorado administers the **CHAMPVA** program. CHAMPVA is not the same entity as CHAMPUS. The Department of Defense manages CHAMPUS, now known as TRICARE.

Dependents (children and spouses) who meet one or more of the following eligibility requirements may qualify for CHAMPVA:

- Veteran has a permanent and total disability that is a service-related disability.
- Veteran died from a VA-related service-connected disability.
- Veteran met the definition of total disability from a service-related disability at the time of death.
- The military member died in the line of duty, and his/her death was not the result of misconduct.
- Note: These individuals will typically qualify for TRICARE and not CHAMPVA.

Due to their veteran status, CHAMPVA sponsors may be entitled to medical treatment through the VA system.

For those who receive Medicare, CHAMPVA is a secondary payer. Those eligible for Medicare must enroll in both Medicare Part A and Medicare Part B to maintain their CHAMPVA benefits.

Models of Care Delivery

There is a wide array of models used to provide care for patients across the continuum of care.

Patient-Centered Medical Home (PCMH)
The **Patient-Centered Medical Home** (PCMH) model provides patients access to comprehensive care. Patients receive access to a well-rounded team of providers ranging from physicians to advanced-practice nurses to physician assistants to nurses, pharmacists, nutritionists, social workers, and care coordinators. The patient is treated as an individual and families are members of the care team, supporting the development and implementation of plans of care.

The PCMH can become a major ally of not only the patient but the case manager as well. The PCMH can assist a patient and his/her family with navigating a complex healthcare-delivery system. They typically provide services that are accessible and offer a variety of communication methods with or on behalf of the patient. This helps patients establish a healthy relationship with their provider and ultimately feel supported during and after business hours.

A physician's practice must pass a set of nine standards and ten must-pass elements to become a designated PCMH. Once a practice achieves recognition, it is viewed as being an organization that follows a core set of principles.

Accountable Care Organization
An **accountable care organization** (ACO) is a network of physicians, hospitals, and other healthcare professionals that purposefully work together to provide adequate care to meet the needs of beneficiaries at a reasonable rate. These organizations are yet another way to assist in managing inefficient payment systems. ACOs can be hospital-led, physician-led, or joint-led.

Currently there are more than 550 Medicare ACOs that serve more than 12 million beneficiaries. There are almost 1000 ACOs currently active and almost half of those are physician-led.

ACOs that are unable to keep costs down or meet performance expectations place themselves at risk for paying penalties or being saddled with additional spending.

Case managers may have a role within ACOs to help keep costs down, but poor performance on the part of the case manager can lead to excessive costs, including the investment made to have them on staff.

The Medicare Shared Savings Program

The Affordable Care Act created the **Medicare Shared Savings Program**. It requires ACOs to hold providers mutually accountable for the health of their patients. They receive financial incentives to cooperate and save money by avoiding services such as diagnostic tests and medical procedures that are not medically necessary.

Pioneer Program

The **Pioneer Program** is another program created by the Centers for Medicare and Medicaid Services (CMS) in which high-performing health systems can keep expected savings as a direct result of accepting greater financial risk.

ACOs may resemble HMOs slightly as it relates to the expected outcomes for patients. There are, however, a few differences. For example, ACO patients are not required to remain in-network, and ACOs have an obligation to meet a set of quality measures to ensure they are not blocking medically necessary care.

Health Home

Health Home was created as a result of the Affordable Care Act of 2010. It is a program that assists in coordinating care for those who suffer from chronic conditions. It is important to note that the Health Home program, a Medicaid program, should not be confused with the Patient-Centered Medical Home (PCMH) model. The PCMH model is sometimes referred to as the "medical home," reflecting that the coordination of care requires a collaborative process between the physician and the individual in need.

Conversely, providers who participate in the Health Home program provide a service that correlates to an integrated clinical approach. Health Homes are responsible for not only coordinating both primary and acute care, but they also must address behavioral health, including substance use disorders and long-term service needs, thus managing and treating the patient holistically. Patients are included in the planning process as required.

The Health Home program delivers care coordination, health promotion, and a comprehensive transition program that includes a care-management package of services. Not only does Home Health identify those services that are available throughout the healthcare-delivery system, but they also seek and make referrals to the community and other social support services.

Health Home providers may be licensed to operate in a variety of settings, including but not limited to a rural health clinic, a community mental-health center, or a home health agency. Also, they may be specialized in a variety of fields; they may be an OB/GYN, or the health home provider may be a group or clinical practice.

Health Homes may consist of a team of varied professionals, including nurses, pharmacists, social workers, or behavioral-health professionals, to name a few. Regardless of background, according to the Centers for Medicaid and Medicare Services, the Home Health team itself should be well-rounded and include medical specialists, nurses, pharmacists, nutritionists, dieticians, social workers, behavioral-health providers, chiropractic professionals, and licensed complementary and alternative practitioners.

Special Needs Plan (SNP)

Special needs plans (SNPs) serve those individuals who suffer from chronic conditions and are recipients of Medicare Part A and Part B. To qualify for an SNP, candidates must reside in the assigned service area.

SNP programs are tailored to meet the needs of those with certain conditions and improve the coordination-of-care process, providing access to hospital care, and medical and prescription-drug benefits, merging them into a single plan.

CMS identifies three groups of SNP recipients:

- **Dual Eligible** (D-SNP). D-SNP recipients have both Medicare and Medicaid.
- **Institutional** (I-SNP). Recipients of I-SNP reside in a nursing home or require nursing care in their home.
- **Chronic Condition** (C-SNP). C-SNP recipients suffer from a severe or disabling condition.

Medicare SNPs have limits on who can participate in their program. A plan may elect only to provide services to those who suffer from diabetes and, thus, build a network of providers who demonstrate a capability of caring for this population in an efficient manner. Also, drug formularies are established in a manner such that they support treatment of those with diabetes.

Under the SNP model, care coordinators may be assigned to support patients along their journey to wellness and to encourage adherence to agreed-upon treatment plan. Support may include education, monitoring of adherence to taking medication, patient empowerment, or providing access to community resources.

Chronic-Care Model (CCM)

More than 130 million people who currently live with a chronic illness live with comorbid conditions. The **chronic-care model** (CCM) is used to support the care given to those suffering from chronic disease. It is a widely accepted and adopted model that is used to improve ambulatory care, and it is a vital player in the Patient-Centered Medical Home model.

CCM consists of four core-strategy concepts: clinical information systems, decision support, delivery-system design, and organizational support. There are two patient-centered concepts in the CCM that form the foundation of this model: self-management support and community resources.

Self-Management Support

Self-management entails empowering the patient to solve problems, make decisions about his/her healthcare, identify potential resources, take actionable steps, and maintain the patient-provider relationship.

Community Resources

It is important that patients gain access to **community resources**. These resources may consist of peer groups that provide support or community partners, such as service organizations, that can provide educational, financial, and medical/behavioral-health resources.

The CCM has been shown to improve outcomes, particularly among individuals who participate in disease-management-based programs. Organizations who participate in CCM-based programs may find there are up-front costs for implementing a CCM program. However, the outcomes and improvement, as they relate to the number of both days hospitalized and ER visits, is visible as a direct result of this model.

Population Health

Population health is an approach to healthcare that focuses on improving the health of an entire population of patients, as opposed to the traditional model which focuses on individual care. Population health spends much of its resources on high-risk patients and preventive and wellness strategies. The goal is to keep high-risk patients healthy and out of hospitals for as long as possible. Disease management is combined with adherence to treatment plans and managed by a population health case manager who helps steer patients through the healthcare continuum. Case managers can proactively check in with patients to understand the reasons why medications are not being taken or appointments are missed. With the rise in Accountable Care Organizations that receive reimbursement based on keeping patient populations healthy, there is a subsequent rise in the need for population health case managers who are willing to advocate for patients and help them transition efficiently through the healthcare system.

Case managers should work to build a referral network for the potential needs of the population of patients that are serviced. Case managers should endeavor to assure that agencies that will be referred to are appropriate and have a contact person. Post referral, case managers should evaluate the referral to see if patients were satisfied and treatment plans were met using that agency.

Negotiation Techniques

Case managers play a critical role within each of the programs identified in that they not only help to coordinate care and treatments to ensure that the patient remains stable, but they also serve as the liaison between the patient and the community or providers. For a patient to be successful with these programs, the case manager has to have a clear understanding of what the objective is for each of these programs, and then advocate on behalf of the client.

Depending on the provider and managed-care contracts, there may be a need for negotiation when it comes to costs or treatment. The case manager may be responsible for negotiating on behalf of the client in order to get the best treatment possible, as well as to lower costs. Negotiation can also be useful in working with patients, families, and/or providers in developing an appropriate treatment plan.

Negotiation is the process of discussion and cooperation in order to get the best possible solution for all parties. This will likely involve compromise on both sides, but the case manager should compromise as little as possible when it comes to the health of the patient. Therefore, it is important that the case manager knows exactly what they are pursuing in the negotiation. This means thorough preparation and a clear knowledge of the client's needs for treatment and reasonable costs to bring to the negotiation table. Being prepared ahead of time will help the case manager know what to settle for as the bottom line.

When it comes to negotiation, the case manager will be more successful if pursuing cooperative or collaborative negotiation rather than competitive or aggressive negotiation. Cooperative negotiation starts with building a relationship of trust with all those involved in the discussion. This comes about through clear, honest, and responsive communication. Communication is not just speaking, but also involves active listening and appropriate body language.

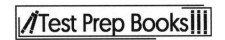

While case managers should be firm in getting what the client needs, they should always conduct the negotiation with respect and a desire to collaborate. Creating an emotionally hostile environment is never helpful, so the case manager should remain calm and de-escalate volatile situations when possible. It is also important to start with areas of common ground and agreement, before moving on to the areas of disagreement. The goal is not to create a situation where one person wins, and one loses. Rather, everyone should come away from the negotiation having gained something.

Physical Functioning and Behavioral-Health Assessment

Physical functioning refers to basic activities of daily life (ADLs), such as eating and bathing. ADLs also include activities that help a person maintain independence, like driving, shopping, or cooking. **Behavioral-health assessments** evaluate a person's level of functioning regarding his/her mental/emotional health, substance abuse, or behavioral needs. These assessments usually use a variety of measures and interview strategies, with both close-ended and open-ended questions that are intended to gather information about the client. While physical functioning and behavioral health may seem unrelated at first glance, they are closely connected to one another.

When it comes to a person's level of physical functioning, there are many factors involved beyond a physical condition or illness. Social and emotional support, mental-health issues such as depression, and a person's cognitive functioning can all contribute to physical functioning. Research has found a correlation between physical functioning and mental health. Many different forms of mental illness can include physical symptoms, such as changes in appetite, sleep disorders, fatigue, and even pain. Though these physical symptoms all contribute to impaired physical functioning, the root cause may be behavioral or mental, rather than physical. When evaluating a client with low physical functioning, it is important to also assess his/her behavioral health. Something like depression may point to a nonphysical cause, such as a lack of motivation or lack of enjoyment in daily activities, which may be hindering the ADLs.

Both physical and mental limitations can have a significant impact on one's quality of life and can lead to an increased risk of falls, bone fractures, depression, and increased healthcare costs. Assessments can help to reveal inadequacies among support systems and allow case managers the opportunity to collaborate with other members of the healthcare-delivery team to address these limitations, whether by way of implementing services, coordinating care, or adjusting treatment plans.

Private Benefit Programs

Consumers have the option to pursue a variety of **private-based benefit programs**.

Pharmacy Benefits Management

Pharmacy-benefits management (PBM) consists of third-party administrators (TPAs) whose primary responsibilities are associated with prescription-drug programs. PBMs work strategically with self-insured companies and government programs to maintain formularies and establish pharmacy contracts. PBM also has a role in negotiating discounts and rebates with pharmaceutical companies. These TPAs earn their revenue as a direct result of service fees that result from large contracts for processing prescription-drug claims. PBM influences more than eighty percent of drug coverage, therefore giving them a significant voice in the healthcare decision-making process.

Indemnity

Indemnity insurance, known as a fee-for-service plan, allows consumers to direct their own healthcare. Customers are able to visit physicians, including specialists, of their choice and are permitted to seek care at the hospital of their choice. A portion of the "total charges" are covered by the insurance company.

Most consumers of this program are required to pay their deductible first, and after this is met the insurance company will pay the claims at a percentage of UCR, also known as the usual, customary, and reasonable rate. Indemnity plans work well for those looking to have the freedom to choose which doctors provide their care and the ability to see the specialist of their choice.

Employer-Sponsored Health Coverage

Many companies offer their employees private health insurance as a component of their benefits package. Sixty percent of Americans obtain health insurance from their employer. Employer-sponsored health-coverage plans are able to provide employees with a variety of options, including vision and dental coverage. In addition, employer-sponsored health-coverage plans are able to provide their employees with short-term and long-term disability, as well as a modest life- insurance policy. These programs may be HMO based, PPO based, or both; thus, employees have the option to choose an HMO or PPO.

Individual-Purchased Insurance

Individuals may purchase insurance for themselves or to cover members of their families instead of relying on coverage offered by an employer. Previously, **individual plans** offered coverage that was less than what is typically seen with group insurance plans. However, as a result of the Affordable Care Act, these plans now include benefits that are more robust.

Home Care Benefits

Insurance may elect to cover **home care services** so that individuals can remain in their home environment as opposed to being placed in a nursing home. Home care agencies can offer a variety of services in the home, especially help with activities of daily living such as bathing, dressing, grooming, and meal preparation.

Many home care services are covered by insurance companies specializing in long-term care; however, recipients must understand if there are any limits for the amount of services that can be received in a single day or over a number of years.

COBRA

Passed in 1986, the **Consolidated Omnibus Reconciliation Act** (COBRA) established a mandate that employers provide their employees with the opportunity to maintain their insurance coverage through the employer in instances in which coverage would typically be terminated. Examples of such loss of insurance would include terminations, layoffs, deaths, Medicare coverage, or other changes in employment status.

Duration of Coverage

The qualifying event defines the length of COBRA coverage.

- Coverage is allowed for up to eighteen months if there is a job termination or reduction in work hours.

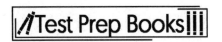

- Coverage is granted for up to twenty-nine months for those individuals who are disabled at any time during the initial sixty days of COBRA coverage.

- Coverage is allowed for up to thirty-six months in instances of death, divorce, legal separation, acquisition of Medicare, a change in a child's dependent status, or other **qualifying events**.

COBRA continuation can be expensive and, therefore, recipients may eventually look for more affordable options. While most group health plans are required to abide by COBRA provisions, employers are exempt from COBRA if they employed fewer than twenty employees during the previous calendar year.

Employers must send a notice to their employee once a **triggering event** takes place. Those who fail to do their due diligence in communicating with the employee put their organization at risk for litigation and create liability for plans.

COBRA Beneficiary Qualifications
An employee's beneficiary may also qualify for COBRA benefits. The **beneficiary** is a covered employee, spouse, dependent, or child of the said covered employee.

COBRA Election Period
Qualified beneficiaries may elect to maintain healthcare coverage from the employer's group health plan through COBRA within sixty days after the date on which plan coverage terminates. If the beneficiary fails to elect COBRA coverage, he/she loses all rights to benefits. There is some flexibility in the selection of COBRA coverage for beneficiaries. Beneficiaries have the ability to choose COBRA coverage independently, and parents can elect COBRA coverage on the behalf of a minor/child.

Coverage
COBRA coverage is equal to the previous insurance plan that the beneficiary received. **COBRA coverage** may include:

- Prescriptions
- Physician visits
- Dental/vision services
- Inpatient and outpatient services

COBRA Payments
Employees or those beneficiaries who qualify for COBRA are required to pay a percentage of administrative costs and the premium.

Public Benefit Programs

Supplemental Security Income (SSI)
Supplemental Security Income (SSI) provides payment of benefits to those individuals and their family members who are living with a limited income and resources (e.g., home, car, land) at their disposal.

Eligible recipients for SSI fall into one or more of the following categories:

- Aged (sixty-five years of age or older)
- Blind
- Disabled

In addition to falling under these three categories and being a US citizen who resides in one of the fifty states, potential recipients must demonstrate that they are of limited income or resources. Next, they must have lived in the United States for a minimum of thirty consecutive days.

Children are also eligible for SSI. To qualify, children under the age of eighteen must exhibit a condition (medical or behavioral) that may:

- Result in death
- Be defined as chronic
- Cause severe functional limitations

Social Security Disability Insurance (SSDI)

Supplemental Security Disability Insurance (SSDI) provides payment of benefits for individuals and their family members if they have worked for enough years and paid Social Security taxes. People who become disabled before the age of retirement can apply for SSDI.

During an individual's lifetime of working, he/she earns four work credits for each year worked. To meet eligibility requirements for SSDI, applicants must have a diagnosis that meets the Social Security Administration's definition of a disability. The disabled condition must fall into the category of:

- **Severe**: A condition that prevents one from performing work-related functions
- **Long term**: A condition that will last greater than twelve months
- **Total disability**: A condition that prevents one from being able to perform SGA, also known as **substantial gainful activity**

Applicants for SSDI will not be approved to receive SSDI until they are disabled for five months. Once approved, there is an opportunity for receipt of retro payment of disability beginning in the sixth month.

Those who have not worked long enough to receive SSDI can apply for SSI.

Medicare

Medicare was established in 1965 to provide healthcare coverage to adults over the age of sixty-five. Since then, the scope of Medicare has changed and now extends to those with disabilities who are younger than age sixty-five who also meet the Social Security Administration's criteria.

Medicare operates in four parts: Part A, Part B, Part C, and Part D.

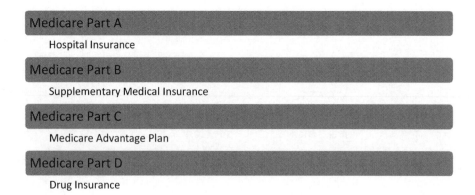

Medicare Part A

Hospital Insurance

Medicare Part B

Supplementary Medical Insurance

Medicare Part C

Medicare Advantage Plan

Medicare Part D

Drug Insurance

Medicare Part A

Medicare Part A, sometimes referred to as Hospital Insurance, covers the hospital portion of healthcare, paying for acute care and skilled-nursing facility (SNF) care.

Medicare Part B

Medicare Part B, also known as Supplementary Medical Insurance, is an optional and additional coverage that pays for physician services, outpatient services, and ancillary charges such as durable medical equipment, preventive services, and some medications. Those who are covered by Part B have premiums deducted from their Social Security income check.

Medicare Part C

Established as a result of the Balanced Budget Act (BBA) of 1997, **Medicare Part C** was created to serve as the Medicare managed care option. Formerly known as **Medicare + Choice Plans** and now known as **Medicare Advantage Plans**, Medicare Part C allows recipients of Medicare to maintain their benefits; however, the managed care organization is chosen and paid by the federal government to administer the Medicare benefits. The MCO may opt to provide coverage for additional services.

Special needs plans deliver managed care services to individuals with special needs such as the chronically ill with conditions such as diabetes, congestive heart failure, or end-stage renal disease. Thus, they specialize in providing managed care that can support complex populations in a cost-effective manner using industry-recognized best practices.

Prescription Drug Plans

Prescription Drug Plans have standards that are dictated by Medicare, although managed by providing companies. While PDPs can provide more than the minimum required package, they can require a higher premium payment for increased coverage. PDPs earn revenue through their facilitation of delivery of prescription medications based on a cost that is less than income.

Medicare Part D provides coverage for those drugs that qualify under the Medicaid program, but this does not include those medications that are available under Part B.

Dual-eligible and low-income Medicare recipients can enroll in PDPs specifically designed for this population where Medicare pays the premium. They do not have to pay a deductible under this program. For those who qualify as indigent, Medicare provides a low-income subsidy that pays costs associated with cost-sharing and premiums.

Medicaid

Title XIX of the Social Security Act of 1965 established the system known as **Medicaid**. Families and individuals who require medical assistance but have limited resources to pay for those services may qualify for Medicaid. Medicaid is co-funded by both the state and federal governments to support the delivery of proper medical care to eligible individuals. State legislatures have the option to re-evaluate and update Medicaid eligibility and services offered during the year. The state government may also adjust reimbursement rates to accommodate trends in healthcare.

States must comply with Medicaid coverage expectations for certain groups to receive federal funds. While states may choose to deliver state-only programs, these are not funded by the federal government. The following mandatory Medicaid categorically needy groups are eligible for government funds:

- Pregnant women with a family income below 133 percent of the federal poverty level (FPL)
- SSI recipients (in most states)
- Those receiving adoption or foster care under Title IV of the Security Act
- Those who qualify for the AFDC or Aid to Families with Dependent Children program
- Children below the age of six whose household income is below 133 percent of the FPL

State programs must offer adequate medical support and services to their categorically needy populations, and those services include:

- Physician services
- Prenatal care
- Outpatient services
- Inpatient services
- Nursing facility services
- Laboratory services
- X-ray services
- Vaccines for children
- Rural health clinics
- Home health
- Skilled-nursing services

States may also elect to extend Medicaid coverage to other populations. These populations may have characteristics that are similar to the mandatory Medicaid recipient groups, but states have greater flexibility to define eligibility criteria for these other populations.

With the implementation of the Affordable Care Act of 2010, states can now choose to extend Medicaid coverage to all low-income Americans under the age of sixty-five. Currently, all but 14 states have extended their program to include this group.

While the federal government provides an overarching set of guidelines, states are responsible for administering their Medicaid programs and defining eligibility standards. The states establish payment rates and are responsible for determining the scope and type of services they wish to make available to recipients, as well as the amount and duration of those services.

Some states can also apply to participate in CMS waiver programs to provide Medicaid services that fall outside of the traditional set of services provided under state Medicaid plans.

Medically Needy

States can establish **Medically Needy** programs to provide access to care for people who earn too much income to qualify for Medicaid. These individuals may become eligible for Medicaid by having expenses that exceed their income and the state's medically needy income level, also known as a **spend down** amount. Once the individual meets this criteria, he or she can have costs for services covered by the Medicaid program.

Employer-based Health and Wellness Programs

Employer-based health and wellness programs have been around for some time with the goal of creating a culture of wellness. The effects of that culture of wellness usually include less absenteeism and lowering the cost of employer-provided health coverage. Many employees enjoy the rewards of the programs, which can include gift cards, contributions toward insurance, and discounts at fitness clubs, amongst other promotions. Programs can either be participatory, where participants earn rewards for participating in activities such as completing a health assessment, or health-contingent, where rewards are impacted by health factors such as being tobacco-free or enrolling in a health coaching program. The Affordable Care Act, the Americans with Disabilities Act, and the Genetic Information Nondiscrimination Act have regulations aimed at protecting patients with health conditions from having their benefits limited due to those conditions. These regulations should prevent employers from requiring employees to take medical exams or mandating them to provide their health information, and may also state that employers cannot require participation in these programs or deny employees coverage access based on participation.

Reimbursement and Payment Methodologies

Case managers may be required to facilitate payments for their organization, as well as monitor for accuracy in billing by a servicing provider. There are several different types of reimbursement and payment methodologies that may be used.

Bundled
In the case of **bundled** payments, providers and healthcare facilities (separately or jointly) may receive a single payment to provide treatment for a condition. Providers assume greater financial risk with this particular payment model. Providers cannot predict what complications may or may not arise as a result of one's diagnosis, but if the actual cost of services proves to be less than the bundled amount there is an opportunity to retain the difference.

In today's landscape of healthcare, the bundled-payment model is used retrospectively. Providers receive payment from the payer once care is complete. Bundled payments may reduce costs while improving care coordination and quality for patients.

Case Rate
Case rates, sometimes referred to as global rates, are pre-negotiated rates put into place for a particular procedure. Case rates ideally include all of the anticipated services that would be required to deliver the treatment.

Prospective Payment System (PPS)
Medicare uses the **Prospective Payment System** (PPS) method of reimbursement. The PPS pays out a preset amount to healthcare providers, which is based on the patient's DRG to approximate the costs of the services provided.

CMS uses a separate PPS for reimbursement for different services on the continuum of care, ranging from inpatient hospitals to psychiatric facilities to long-term care facilities.

Value-Based Purchasing (VBP)

The **Value-Based Purchasing** (VBP) program is an initiative utilized by CMS to persuade acute-care hospitals to provide quality-based care to Medicare beneficiaries through the use of incentive-based payments. This process involves close monitoring of how well hospitals follow best clinical practices. Hospitals also receive an evaluation for how well they can improve the patients' hospital stay experience.

CMS monitors hospital performance by using a set of measures and dimensions, which are grouped into specific quality-driven domains.

Measuring Hospital Total Performance

CMS evaluates the hospital's **total-performance** score, which compares achievement and improvement scores for each of the hospital's Value-Based Purchasing measures. The Achievement Points awarded to a hospital are directly tied to the comparison of an individual hospital's rates during a performance period with that of all hospitals' rates from a specified baseline period.

Improvement Points are granted based on a comparison of an individual hospital's ratings to its ratings during the baseline period.

Consistency Points are granted through a comparison of the hospital's HCAHPS base score and the hospital's HCAHPS consistency score.

Financial Risk Models

Under traditional payment models, providers were paid for services performed. After the ACA came into play, more alternative payment models were introduced. Under these alternative payment models, providers become financially responsible for the care given. In upside risk (sometimes called one-sided risk), providers receive a share of the savings when they save money by providing more efficient care but are not penalized if they do not meet the benchmark. With downside risk (also known as two-sided risk), providers can receive a share of savings but can also lose revenue if the healthcare they provide doesn't financially meet the benchmark. Most ACOs who use alternative payment models prefer to only use the upside risk model. To hold more ACOs financially accountable, CMS has made Tracks for ACOs participating. Many of the tracks now require a three year contract which includes a downside risk period after only an upside risk initially. The shift to allow more providers to use downside risk models is necessary for ACOs to be successful in saving money in overall care. More work must be done in building out post-acute care and preventive care to make alternative models and their financial risk models more appealing to providers.

Roles and Functions of Case Managers in Various Care/Practice Settings

Case management may take place in any setting throughout the care continuum. Case managers may work in a wide variety of settings, including hospitals, disease-management organizations, MCOs, ACOs, prisons, hospice organizations, independent case-management services, and corporations, to name a few.

Acute-Care Settings

Case managers who use the case-management process in an acute-care setting are required to support the hospital in providing care that is adequate and cost-effective.

Therefore, the goal of a case manager in an **acute-care setting** might include:

- Monitoring for a change in the level of care such that it is a lesser but appropriate level of care
- Monitoring for a reduction in the length of stay based on industry or organization guidelines for care
- Ensuring the delivery of those services that are medically necessary

Managed Care Settings

Managed care case managers, who are sometimes referred to as internal and/or external case managers working for a payer-based system, look to support the MCO's mission and goals, which may include but are not limited to a reduction of:

- The number of inpatient admissions
- The duration or length of hospital stays
- Delays in discharge to home with adequate home care services

Government Settings

Case managers may operate in **government settings,** including government-operated healthcare facilities and Health and Human Services. Due to their background and experiences, case managers may also support activities such as research and administrative tasks. Case managers may also work in settings in which they assist with grant writing, program development and implementation.

Home Health Care

Case managers who work in the **Home Health Care setting** are responsible for ensuring the safety of the environment for the patient. A comprehensive assessment is performed by a case manager to evaluate the patient's functional needs and the patient's ability to transfer from a hospital setting to a home environment. Comprehensive assessments can also assist in determining whether or not the patient or caregiver can provide adequate care. Much of the home care facilitated by case managers encompasses education and health progression.

Case managers who work for home healthcare agencies are provider-based case managers. **Provider-based** case managers work within organizations and facilities such as IPAs, rehabilitation centers, hospitals, and behavioral-healthcare locations.

For long-term illnesses, case managers may be required to assist families with enlisting attendant care or respite-care services where applicable and available.

Community-based case managers are those case managers who work with nonprofit agencies as well as local state departments. Their core population consists of those communities that are low income or Medicaid and Medicare recipients.

Roles and Functions of Other Healthcare Providers in Various Care/Practice Settings

Providers from **various settings** may be used throughout the continuum of care and to support case-management activities. Interdisciplinary teams are made up of many different types of providers, ensuring that the patient is getting the care needed in every area of life and functioning. It is important for the case manager to understand the role and function of each provider in order to most effectively coordinate the care the patient receives.

Many of these providers will be medical practitioners, such as doctors, nurse practitioners, nurses, nurse midwives, speech or physical therapists, and various specialists. General medical practitioners, such as doctors and nurse practitioners, will oversee the patient's medical care. A patient is likely to have a primary-care physician, who has the job of managing the patient's general health and referring to other specialists. Depending on the patient's condition, there may also be other specialists involved, like oncologists, dieticians, chiropractors, surgeons, or cardiologists. Even professionals such as dentists or pharmacists may play a crucial role in the process of treatment. Some of the primary responsibilities fulfilled by these medical practitioners are diagnosis of the disease, prescription of medicines, surgeries and other treatments, and monitoring of the patient's overall health status.

Psychologists, psychiatrists, social workers, and therapists may also be involved in care to address the mental-health needs of the patient. Psychologists can conduct psychological evaluations or behavioral-health assessments to provide a more complete understanding of the patient's overall well-being. Therapists can provide counseling that a patient may need to deal with issues of anxiety, depression, or other mental illness that may occur as a result of dealing with acute or chronic illness. Psychiatrists typically prescribe mental-health medications for the patient. When a case manager is coordinating treatment for a patient, both the mental health and physical health must be fully understood and treated, as they can have a great impact on each other.

Along with medical practitioners and mental-health providers, the patient may have others involved in treatment, whether through community resources or informal providers, such as family or caregivers. This might include support groups that may be led by peers, home health aides, or organizations providing disease-specific financial aid or education. While these providers may not have a direct role in guiding medical care, they are certainly significant when it comes to the client's social, financial, and emotional well-being, which can all impact health.

While every patient is different and will require a unique combination of providers, one of the tasks of the case manager is to evaluate whether a patient is receiving the necessary treatment, through the most appropriate providers. It is also important to remember that at the center of the decision-making team is the patient, and he/she should never be overlooked when treatment options and plans are being discussed among the professionals.

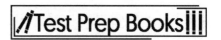

Transitions of Care/Transitional Care

The **transition of care** involves the movement of patients within and between various settings and providers. This change in the level of care is driven by a change in the patient's condition and medical or behavioral-health needs.

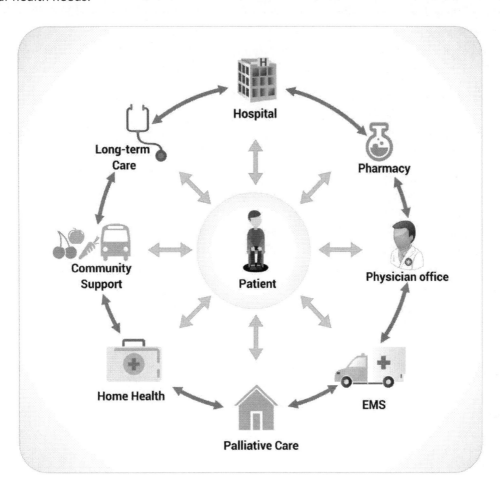

Successful transitions require effective care coordination and logistical planning to reduce the risk of health complications that could lead to readmissions, adverse events, an increase in healthcare costs, or a greater length of stay.

Open communication between highly trained practitioners and healthcare professionals and the patient/caregiver must take place to reduce the risk of an adverse health outcome for the patient. Good communication requires a comprehensive plan of care and collaboration between healthcare providers, who should all be made aware of the patient's goals, preferences, and clinical status. A successful transition plan includes scheduling and keeping follow-up appointments, home visits, and effective medication management, which includes ongoing medication reconciliation.

The purpose of the **National Transitions of Care Coalition** (NTOCC) is to address the problems associated with transitions of care.

The NTOCC recommends the following:

- Payment systems that align incentives
- Implementation of performance measures to encourage or/improve transitions of care
- Increased utilization of case-management services
- Utilization of pharmacists during the transition of care process as it relates to medication reconciliation

Utilization Management Principles and Guidelines

Utilization-management (UM) functions act as a predecessor to case management in many organizations. In fact, it often operates as a separate entity, determining the medical necessity for hospital admissions and procedures. It also determines the appropriateness of the assigned level of care.

UM clinicians act as stewards of insurance companies and other payers' dollars, using organization-specific criteria such as critical pathways and clinical guidelines, and industry-recognized criteria like McKesson InterQual or Milliman, to review the medical necessity of hospital care. UM clinicians can identify that the level of care is inappropriate based on the patient's clinical presentation. However, UM clinicians and medical directors must also use their clinical expertise and judgment to allow for medically necessary treatment even when, clinically, a patient's presentation does not fully align to the criteria sets.

UM clinicians work closely with case managers to not only gain a full picture of the patient but also to allow for continuity of care during the discharge-planning process.

Unlike case management, utilization management is more episodic in nature, and centers on the hospitalization and length of stay of a patient for an illness. Case management spans the continuum of care, following the patient throughout the various healthcare settings and back into his/her home environment.

Organizations who facilitate the utilization review process may apply for accreditation via the **Utilization Review Accreditation Commission** (URAC). URAC establishes standards and guidelines by which UM entities can evaluate themselves. These measures include the use of evidence-based guidelines, the level of review requirements for reviewers, and policies that address financial incentives given to providers.

Collaborative/Comprehensive/Integrated/Holistic Case Management Services

As healthcare continues to change, the role of the case manager continues to change. The shift to integrated and holistic case management is at the forefront of that change. The integrated case management process begins with the case manager developing a genuine relationship with a patient, and considering together with the patient their goals, concerns, and needs. Integrated and holistic case management processes are especially important for patients who are medically complex. Using this process involves using appropriate assessment tools from the start, once a relationship is established. A commonly used tool for assessment is the ICM-CAG (Integrated Case Management Complexity Assessment Grid). This assessment tool assists the case manager to use a color coded system to determine the levels of risks that the patient is facing, so that together the patient and case manager can address the immediate risks. This type of collaborative and integrated approach is especially important for patients that face behavioral and mental health struggles in addition to medical issues.

Chronic conditions, such as heart disease or hypertension, become more difficult to manage when combined with mental illness and can lead to poor outcomes. Case managers who with the integrated process see treating the patient as a whole as leading to better outcomes and help coordinate many types of services for an individual patient.

Caseload Considerations

In order to ensure that each case receives suitable and efficient attention, it is essential that all cases are assigned according to acuity. **Caseload calculations** allow for what equates to an appropriate volume of clients for case managers, while demonstrating the case managers' ability to provide quality case management services. The periodic tabulation of the caseload of any specific case manager is integral to combat inconsistencies within and among organizations. According to the **Caseload Concept Paper** published by the Case Management Society of America (CMSA) and the National Association of Social Workers (NASW) in 2008, the average caseload for case managers was in a range of 2 to 365. This study led to the creation of the **Case Load Capacity Calculator** by the CMSA and NASW in collaboration with Consulting Management Innovators. The free calculator enables teams to calculate comparative caseload capacities within case management departments for the domain the case manager is supporting; disseminates industry-based rules and weights (e.g., time allocation for various activities, complexity of the case, environmental factors/settings); and allows for caseload customization by creating a baseline for how cases are distributed.

The **Caseload Matrix** is a diagram, also known as a schematic chart, that is divided into four categories. Provided by the CMSA and the NASW Concept Paper, the matrix interprets those facets known to have an impact on the size and complexity of a caseload. Each of the four categories has elements that define the complex nature of a caseload and caseload size. Based on these four variables, case assignment is more efficient and equitable. Below are the caseload matrix categories. They provide an overview of how each category is defined and which elements align with each of these categories.

Any change in a factor of this chart has a direct impact on other categories and any associated elements. Case managers who follow their patients throughout the continuum of healthcare must monitor their caseloads closely for changes that affect acuity. Utilizing the matrix will alert the case manager to changes in acuity and adjust case assignment in an effort to be proactive instead of being reactive.

Alternative Care Sites

Non-Traditional Sites of Care

As the role of case management continues to evolve, non-traditional sites of care continue to emerge. Case managers find themselves working more in long-term care: provider's offices, insurance companies, surgery centers, mobile medical units, and shelters. Being able to work from these non-traditional sites of care means that instead of a case manager's job ending when a patient leaves the hospital, it is just beginning. With most non-traditional sites, the goal becomes keeping patients at their maximum level of health and decreasing hospitalizations. As the emphasis on population health increases, due in part to the goals of Healthy People 2020, case managers are likely to find their roles in these non-traditional sites of care more valuable than ever.

Telehealth

Technology is improving access to healthcare for many patients. Today, telehealth (also referred to as telemedicine) refers to patient care that happens without being in-person. Telehealth is especially useful for non emergent, chronic illnesses. Telehealth is emerging as a way to optimize revenue for providers and increase patient satisfaction. Many patients prefer not to drive to a location and wait to access healthcare. Telehealth growth happened much quicker than expected in many types of healthcare, including case management due to COVID-19. Telehealth is considered useful at expanding access to healthcare while keeping patients safe. At times, a patient will seek telehealth and be told that they need to seek in-person care because they can not be safely treated via telehealth.

Virtual Care

Virtual care is a broader term than telehealth and describes the many different types of healthcare services that can be done virtually (including telehealth). Virtual care may refer to anything from electronic vital sign monitoring to responding via messenger to a patient's question. Virtual care includes reviewing the EHR, using wearable technology, and even using healthcare apps. Revenue can be optimized using virtual care, especially in alternative payment models, where keeping patients healthy and out of hospitals leads to more sharing in financial savings by ACOs. Case managers may find themselves using virtual care to engage with patients at high risk for not adhering to treatment plans. Discovering reasons for their non adherence may help case managers direct patients to other forms of virtual care that keep patients at optimal levels of health. As more ACOs with their alternative payment models enter the system, case managers' roles will likely change, with much of their job just beginning when the patient is discharged from the hospital, as they use all these virtual care resources to keep the patient adhering to their plan of care, and out of the hospital, thus maximizing financial sharing.

Practice Questions

1. Which of the following is NOT a cause of nonadherence to the care regimen?
    a. Financial limitations
    b. Limited understanding of an illness or condition
    c. Positive reinforcement of positive behavior
    d. Poor health literacy

2. Which of the following is true of adult foster care?
    a. May be used as an alternative to institutionalized living in some states
    b. Managed by volunteer caregivers
    c. Is unable to provide support for activities of daily living
    d. May not be used for the elderly

3. Which of the following is true about residential treatment services?
    a. May be provided for an indeterminate amount of time
    b. Can provide patients with greater access to services that are more intensive than outpatient services
    c. May not be used for mental illness, substance abuse, or other behavioral-health needs
    d. Do not offer case managers a role during the time a patient is admitted to a residential treatment facility.

4. Which of the following is true about group homes?
    a. They are not staffed twenty-four hours per day
    b. They do not provide a permanent alternative living solution for adults over the age of nineteen
    c. They may be used for those suffering from a chronic mental illness or dementia
    d. They are set up as non-profit businesses

5. What is true of assessments done during the case-management process?
    a. Intended to only be completed once during the lifecycle of a case
    b. Not a one-time event but may be repeated to establish and/or monitor ongoing needs throughout the case-management process
    c. Only able to yield information about the physical background but not the psychosocial aspect of a patient's health
    d. Not intended to be a part of the initial steps taken by a case manager in the case-management process but rather a supplementary action item that can be done at any time during the process

6. What should happen during the planning phase of the case-management process?
    a. Case managers must work in a solo-fashioned format to ensure that a robust plan of care is developed and medically acceptable to all healthcare providers responsible for providing care
    b. Case managers must leave goals as originally written despite changes in the patient's priority that may occur throughout the case-management process
    c. Case managers must ensure that there are not multiple interventions for every goal
    d. Case managers may modify goals during the case-management process due to barriers or complications that arise, but these goals should remain individualized and specific to the patient and monitored closely with a secondary or alternative plan in place

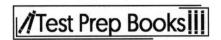

7. What is important for the case manager to consider when developing care plans?
    a. Do not require approval by anyone except the case manager
    b. Should only be reviewed by the patient and the case manager
    c. Should only be reviewed by the case manager and treating provider
    d. Should capture ongoing progress of the client as well as any barriers that are preventing adherence to care

8. Which of the following is NOT included in an intervention that is executed during the intervention phase?
    a. Case manager educates a client about the appropriate A1C levels
    b. Case manager requests an authorization for a home health safety assessment
    c. Case manager coordinates transportation for a client to his/her next specialist visit
    d. Case manager cancels follow-up call to client

9. When can case managers close a case?
    a. When the patient has not yet fully demonstrated adherence to care
    b. When services are in place to sufficiently meet the needs of the patient
    c. When the patient demonstrates an ability to seek healthcare support through the appropriate channels
    d. B & C.

10. Which of the following is used by mental-health professionals and other healthcare professionals, including case managers, to classify mental illness?
    a. Diagnostic and Statistical Manual of Mental Disorders
    b. International Classification of Diseases
    c. Diagnosis-Related Groups
    d. Current Procedural Terminology

11. Which of the following is a medical code that is utilized along with ICD numerical diagnostic coding as a component of the billing process?
    a. Hospital Illness-Related Diagnosis
    b. Medical Terminology Coding
    c. Diagnosis-Related Groups
    d. Current Procedural Terminology

12. Which of the following is a standard diagnostic tool that is leveraged to track epidemiology and support health management and clinical activities?
    a. International Coding of Disorders
    b. International Classification of Diseases
    c. International Disease Terminology
    d. International Procedural Terminology

13. Which of the following are used to group patients based on their diagnosis and type of treatment, including surgical procedures along with the presence or absence of comorbidities or complications?
    a. Disease-specific groups
    b. Illness-classification systems
    c. Diagnosis-related groups
    d. Disease-grouping systems

14. Which of the following happens from birth to the start of an illness to the point in which the patient is either no longer ill or the patient is no longer eligible for medical or case-management services?
    a. Continuing Spectrum of Care
    b. Case Management Continuum
    c. Continuum Alliance
    d. Continuum of Care

15. What is an activity of case management that can contribute to cost containment?
    a. Identifying barriers to care
    b. Finding coupons for the client
    c. Keeping phone calls to a minimum
    d. Canceling doctor's visits on behalf of the client

16. Which of the following regarding acuity levels is NOT true?
    a. They can inform decisions made regarding the case-management model used by an organization and the staffing levels necessary to support their programs.
    b. They can assist both case managers and departments in monitoring a case manager's caseload and ensuring the case manager maintains a proper caseload mix.
    c. Data gained during the initial intake screening and the level of services the patient will require over a short-term period can aid in assigning the patient's acuity level.
    d. They are established by the national acuity model that is utilized by all healthcare-delivery systems

17. What may be sold by an individual who is facing a terminal illness to relieve financial burdens and occurs when an individual elects to sell his/her life-insurance policy?
    a. Terminal illness settlements
    b. Viatical settlements
    c. Waiver settlements
    d. Contract settlements

18. What are designed to support those who lack the mental capacity to manage their own finances?
    a. Special needs trusts
    b. Disability trust funds
    c. Special needs assistance
    d. Special assistance trusts

19. Which of the following are a combination of standard medical and nonmedical services that may allow for the provision of long-term care services in the home and community?
    a. Combo service assistance programs
    b. Home health promotion programs
    c. Waiver programs
    d. Contract establishment programs

20. Which of the following are NOT goals of case management?
    a. Provide service and care coordination
    b. Promote care that is medically necessary and cost-effective
    c. Create a pathway to functional stability
    d. Impose the case manager's values onto the client

21. Behavioral-health providers include which of the following?
    a. Physical therapists
    b. Childcare workers
    c. Psychologists
    d. Nurses

22. Which of the following may be administered at any stage of an illness or at any age on behalf of their patient?
    a. Hospice care
    b. End-of-life services
    c. Guideline-based healing care
    d. Palliative care

23. What is typically administered as a component of end-of-life care to those who are suffering from terminal illnesses with less than six months to live?
    a. Hospice care
    b. Critical pathway care
    c. Chronic illness care
    d. Palliative care

24. When should a case manager look for end-of-life care issues to be discussed?
    a. At the end of life
    b. After treatment begins
    c. Only at the request of the patient
    d. Early on in the decision-making process

25. Which of the following is administered over a period of time not to exceed two years?
    a. Long-term disability
    b. Accidental insurance
    c. Short-term disability
    d. Long-term care services

26. What is used to replace the income lost as a result of a chronic condition or illness?
    a. Long-term disability
    b. Chronic-condition insurance
    c. Long-term Social Security
    d. Long-term care services

27. In what way do workers' compensation case managers assist the insurance payer?
    a. By communicating with the doctors so they know when the patient is to return to work
    b. By formulating the most effective treatment plan
    c. By reporting the status and progress of the patient's treatment
    d. By determining when the patient can return to work

28. What is an interdisciplinary care team?
    a. A collaborative group of healthcare professionals from different backgrounds, disciplines, and professions
    b. A group of doctors that collaborate together in treating an illness
    c. A community group of peer support for the client
    d. A group of family members and friends hand-picked by the client to support them

29. Which of the following is considered a form of long-term care?
    a. Emergency care
    b. Assisted living
    c. Outpatient clinic
    d. Vocational training

30. An insurance company sets a limit of $50,000 as the total cost that they will cover in claims, with the remaining costs above $50,000 and up to $500,000 being covered by another carrier. What is this carrier known as?
    a. Reinsurance or stop-loss carrier
    b. Health-insurance extension coverage
    c. Viatical settlement
    d. Viatical trust

31. Which of the following requires ACOs to hold providers mutually accountable for the health of their patients, providing them with financial incentives to cooperate and save money by avoiding services such as diagnostic tests and medical procedures that are not medically necessary?
    a. Pioneer Program
    b. Medicaid Shared Savings Program
    c. ACO Shared Savings Program
    d. Medicare Shared Savings Program

32. Which of the following does NOT require referral to see a specialist, nor has a requirement to choose a primary-care physician?
    a. HMO
    b. IPA
    c. PPO
    d. POS

33. Which of the following is required by the Affordable Care Act to manage a minimum of 5,000 Medicare beneficiaries for a period of five years?
    a. HMOs
    b. IPAs
    c. PPOs
    d. ACOs

34. What is the main difference between acute and chronic illnesses?
    a. Duration of the illness
    b. Severity of the illness
    c. Medication regimen
    d. Mental health of the patient

35. Which of the following were established with the US Medicare Modernization Act of 2003 for the primary purpose of promoting medication adherence among Medicare Part D beneficiaries through the use of education and counseling?
    a. Medicare Therapy Management Program
    b. Medication Therapy Management Program
    c. Medicare Therapy Modernization Program
    d. Medication Therapy Modernization Program

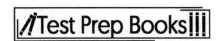

36. Which of the following serves those individuals who suffer from a chronic condition currently receiving Medicare Part A and Part B?
    a. SNP
    b. DNP
    c. PCM
    d. MGP

37. Which of the following provides active-duty family members who have a qualifying mental or physical disability with financial assistance?
    a. TRICARE Disability
    b. TRICARE Special Services
    c. ECHO
    d. SNP

38. Which of the following are NOT eligible for TRICARE?
    a. Medicare Part A recipients
    b. US Family Health Plan participants
    c. Medicare Part B recipients
    d. CHAMPVA recipients

39. Which of the following are responsible for not only coordinating both primary and acute care, but they also must address behavioral health, including substance use disorders, and long-term service needs, thus managing and treating the patient holistically?
    a. Health Homes
    b. Patient-Centered Medical Homes
    c. Long-term care homes
    d. Behavioral treatment homes

40. What must a physician's practice pass to function as a Patient-Centered Medical Home?
    a. Standards and guidelines
    b. Criteria and pathways
    c. Tests and practice guidelines
    d. Standards and elements

41. How can case managers promote self-management in patients?
    a. Limiting the decisions patients make about their own health
    b. Solving problems for the patient
    c. Allowing patients to take actionable steps about their own health
    d. Restricting the patient-provider relationship

42. What is the most effective form of negotiation for the case manager to engage in?
    a. Aggressive negotiation
    b. Collaborative negotiation
    c. Passive negotiation
    d. Simplistic negotiation

43. What does the term *physical functioning* refer to?
    a. A client's level of physical mobility
    b. The amount of exercise engaged in on a daily basis
    c. Physical strength
    d. Activities of daily life, such as eating and bathing

44. Which of the following is true about pharmacy benefits management programs?
    a. work strategically with self-insured companies and government programs to maintain formularies and establish pharmacy contracts.
    b. do not have a role negotiating discounts or rebates with pharmaceutical companies.
    c. have minimal influence over drug coverage.
    d. do not have an active role in prescription-drug programs.

45. Within how many days may qualified beneficiaries elect to maintain healthcare coverage from the employer's group health plan through COBRA?
    a. thirty
    b. forty-five
    c. sixty
    d. ninety

46. Which of the following provides payment of benefits to those individuals and their family members who are living with a limited income and/or resources at their disposal?
    a. SSI
    b. SSDI
    c. FSA
    d. Medicaid

47. Which of the following allows recipients of Medicare to maintain their benefits; however, a managed care organization is chosen and paid by the federal government to administer the Medicare benefits?
    a. Medicare Part A
    b. Medicare Part B
    c. Medicare Part C
    d. Medicare Part D

48. Sometimes referred to as Hospital Insurance, what covers the hospital portion of healthcare, paying for acute care and care at skilled-nursing facilities?
    a. Medicare Part A
    b. Medicare Part B
    c. Medicare Part C
    d. Medicare Part D

49. Which of the following programs provide for those individuals who have significant health needs but whose income is too high to qualify for Medicaid?
    a. Medically needy
    b. Special needs
    c. Patient-Centered Medical Home
    d. Health Home

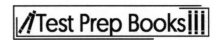

50. Which of the following allows benefits for individuals and their family members if they have worked for enough years to receive Social Security taxes and become disabled prior to the age of retirement?
    a. Medicare
    b. Medicaid
    c. SSI
    d. SSDI

51. Which of the following is true about COBRA requirements?
    a. Employers to terminate insurance coverage upon loss of employment
    b. Employers to provide coverage for up to forty-eight months if job termination is due to disability
    c. Employers to allow their employees the opportunity to maintain their insurance coverage through the employer for up to thirty-six months when the loss of coverage is due to death or divorce
    d. Employers to allow their employees to maintain their insurance coverage through the employer for up to thirty-six months when the loss of coverage is due to job termination or reduction in work hours

52. Which of the following is a reimbursement method that relies on a single payment given to healthcare providers to conduct treatment?
    a. Case rate
    b. Bundled
    c. Prospective payment system
    d. Value-based purchasing

53. Which of the following is NOT included in a successful transition plan?
    a. Keeping appointments
    b. Adhering to medication orders and ongoing medication management and reconciliation
    c. Case-manager goals and preferences
    d. Utilization of home visits for education and assessments

54. Case managers who work for home healthcare agencies are considered which of the following?
    a. Health-progression case managers
    b. Long-term illness case managers
    c. Provider-based case managers
    d. Community-based case managers

55. Which of the following is true about MCO case managers?
    a. Focus more on those populations that require complex management and are at the greatest risk for catastrophic outcomes
    b. Provide services to large percentages of their population
    c. Are not in a favorable position to align themselves with providers and patients
    d. Do not use best practices and guidelines proposed by NCQA

Answer Explanations

1. C: A lack of positive reinforcement of positive behavior by the interdisciplinary healthcare team can contribute to increased nonadherence. Financial limitations, limited understanding of an illness or condition, and poor health literacy can also contribute to increased nonadherence.

2. A: Much like long-term care support services, adult foster care provides support for activities of daily living and provides room and board for the elderly. In some states, it is offered as a component of long-term care waiver programs. It is managed by sponsoring families and paid caregivers.

3. B: Residential treatment services are utilized when outpatient treatment is no longer the most effective approach to treating patients. Residential treatment facilities provide access to fully integrated, long-term, intensive, treatment driven services.

4. C: Group homes provide an alternative living environment for children and adults that is staffed twenty-four hours per day with operational staff. Group homes are for-profit businesses.

5. B: Assessments are not a one-time event. They may be repeated more than once to establish and/or monitor ongoing needs throughout the case-management process. Assessments form the foundation for activities associated with planning, implementation, care coordination, evaluation, and outcomes management.

6. D: The prioritization of goals may change throughout the lifecycle of a case as a patient's focus may also change due to barriers or specific needs. The case-management process is a collaborative process that can utilize multiple interventions to address a single goal.

7. D: Care plans are evolving documents that should be updated throughout the lifecycle of a case to reflect the ongoing progress of the patient. Care plans should be designed and collaborated on by the patient, payer, treating physician, and any others indicated.

8. D: Follow-up calls are an example of an intervention that is performed by a case manager who may frequently maintain contact with a patient to ensure interventions are proving to be effective. Education, request for authorization, and coordinating transportation are other activities often included in the intervention phase.

9. D: Cases should only be closed when certain criteria are demonstrated within the life cycle of a case. Once services are sufficiently in place to support continued improvement or stability of a patient and the patient demonstrates the ability to independently obtain appropriate health status, the case closure is an appropriate next step.

10. A: The DSM is used by mental-health professionals and other healthcare professionals, including case managers, to classify mental illness, as well as for data-collection and billing purposes.

11. D: CPT codes are used to help identify medical, surgical, and diagnostic procedures and services to entities such as physicians, health-insurance companies, and accreditation organizations.

12. B: ICD codes are leveraged to track epidemiology, support health management and to support clinical activities.

13. C: DRGs are used to group patients based on their diagnosis and type of treatment, including surgical procedure along with the presence or absence of comorbidities or complications. Hospital stays are assigned a DRG.

14. D: In case management, patients are at greatest risk during the transition points of care—specifically, when they are transitioning from one level of care to another. The continuum of care (CoC) requires case management of patients in multiple settings. It happens from birth to the start of an illness to the point at which the patient is either no longer ill or the patient is no longer eligible for medical or case-management services.

15. A: If the case manager can identify barriers to care then services will become more effective, ultimately reducing the need for additional services and the costs that will be incurred.

16. D: Case-managed patients are generally assigned an acuity level rating that indicates the severity of an illness or disability, such that case managers can use the acuity level to identify how sick the patient is at the time of case-management engagement. They can inform decisions made regarding the case-management model used by an organization, and the staffing levels necessary to support their programs. Acuity levels can assist both case managers and departments in monitoring a case manager's caseload and ensuring the case manager maintains a proper caseload mix with an equal distribution of cases per acuity level. Data gained during the initial intake screening coupled with the level of services required by the patients over a short-term period can aid in establishing the assigned acuity level for a patient. Currently, there is no standing acuity model or program that is utilized by all healthcare-delivery systems, but rather acuity levels are assigned using various models, software, tools, and resources that have been established by the organization for which the case manager works.

17. B: Viatical settlements are used during a terminal illness to relieve financial burdens. An individual can choose to sell his or her life-insurance policy for a percentage of the face value.

18. A: Specifically, special needs trusts are designed to benefit the disabled or mentally ill. SNTs are designed to support those who lack the mental capacity to manage their own finances.

19. C: Waiver programs may include case management, home health aide, personal attendant care services, adult day health services, respite care, and residential care. On occasion, states may choose to include additional value-added services.

20. D: It is not the job of the case manager to impose his/her value system onto the client. Rather, the case manager should empower the client in self-directed care and support the client's priorities even when contrary to those of the case manager.

21. C: While physical therapists, childcare workers, and nurses may all be providers or involved in the client's life, it is the psychologist that focuses on behavioral health or mental health.

22. D: The characteristic that distinguishes palliative care from hospice care is the time at which palliative care may be offered. Case managers may advocate for palliative care to be administered at any stage of an illness or at any age on behalf of their patient.

23. A: The goal in providing hospice care is not to provide a cure but to ensure that the patient's remaining days are as comfortable as possible.

24. D: This should be discussed early on in the decision-making process since having a plan in place makes the patient's wishes clear and reduces the level of stress for the individual, the family, and the patient.

25. C: Short-term disability is not intended to be long term. There are a set of benefits leveraged to provide coverage for an individual during a time in which they are deemed disabled.

26. A: As the label indicates, long-term disability is used for chronic conditions with the intention of replacing income that is lost as a result of a chronic condition or illness.

27. C: Ultimately, case managers function as objective third parties in workers' compensation cases, using their unique qualifications and experience with medical, social, and vocational issues to advocate for the needs of the patient while reporting relevant information back to the insurance company. They also function as liaison between medical providers, the patient, and the payer. While ensuring the patient is receiving all the care he or she needs, the case manager must also report all information to the insurance adjuster, such as the patient's noncompliance with the treatment program or participation in activities that could delay a return to work. The other listed options are not functions of the case manager alone; they are either determined by the patient's other medical providers or as the entire team working with the patient.

28. A: What is unique about the interdisciplinary care team is that it consists of professionals from many different backgrounds, including nurses, doctors, social workers, dieticians, and family members. They all work together in order to best meet the needs of the client and develop an effective plan of care.

29. B: Assisted living is considered a form of long-term care because it assists those who struggle to care for themselves and to function independently.

30. A: Reinsurance, also known as stop-loss insurance, is a method used to reduce risk or net liability or loss in catastrophic cases that could put an insurance company at risk for losing an amount of money that is so significant that it could cause them to go bankrupt.

31. D: Under the Affordable Care Act, ACOs and providers are mutually accountable for the health of their patients. They receive financial incentives to cooperate and save money by avoiding services such as diagnostic tests and medical procedures that are not medically necessary.

32. C: PPOs are more flexible than HMOs and do not require referrals as seen with other programs.

33. D: This is a component of the ACO framework. Currently, more than 12 million Medicare beneficiaries are enrolled in an ACO.

34. A: The main difference between acute and chronic illnesses is duration, acute being short term and chronic being long term. Treatment for acute illnesses usually focuses on curing the illness, whereas treatment for chronic illnesses is more focused on managing symptoms.

35. B: This is the definition of the Medication Therapy Management Program. Medication Therapy Management Programs (MTMP) were established with the US Medicare Modernization Act of 2003 for the primary purpose of promoting medication adherence among Medicare Part D beneficiaries through the use of education and counseling.

36. A: SNPs are available in specific regions/service areas. Special needs plans (SNP) serve those individuals who suffer from a chronic condition and are recipients of Medicare Part A and Part B.

37. C: This is the purpose of the Extended Care Health Option under the TRICARE program.

38. D: TRICARE and CHAMPVA are two distinct programs.

39. A: Health Home programs are targeted to those who suffer from chronic conditions and expand their scope to include behavioral health and substance-abuse issues.

40. D: A physician's practice must pass a set of nine standards and ten must-pass elements to become a designated PCMH.

41. C: Self-management entails empowering the patient to solve problems and make decisions about his/her healthcare, identifying potential resources, taking actionable steps, and maintaining the patient-provider relationship.

42. B: Collaborative negotiation is the most effective form of negotiation in the case-management context. It is built on relationships of trust and seeks to have everyone come away from the negotiation having gained something.

43. D: Physical functioning refers to basic activities of daily life (ADLs), such as eating and bathing. ADLs also include the activities that help a person maintain independence, like driving, shopping, or cooking. Physical functioning and behavioral health can be closely related.

44. A: PBMs work strategically with self-insured companies and government programs to maintain formularies and establish pharmacy contracts. PBMs also have a role in negotiating discounts and rebates with pharmaceutical companies.

45. C: Within sixty days, qualified beneficiaries may elect to maintain healthcare coverage from the employer's group health plan through COBRA within sixty days after the date in which plan coverage terminates. If the beneficiary fails to elect COBRA coverage, they lose all rights to benefits.

46. A: Supplemental Security Income (SSI) provides payment of benefits to those individuals and their family members who are living with a limited income and resources (e.g., home, car, land) at their disposal.

47. C: Established as a result of the Balanced Budget Act (BBA) of 1997, Medicare Part C was created to serve as the Medicare managed care option.

48. A: Medicare Part A, sometimes referred to as Hospital Insurance, covers the hospital portion of healthcare, paying for acute care and skilled-nursing facility care.

49. A: States may establish *medically needy* programs to provide access to care for people who earn too much income to qualify for Medicaid.

50. D: Supplemental Security Disability Insurance (SSDI) provides payment of benefits for individuals and their family members if they have worked for enough years to receive Social Security taxes. People who become disabled before the age of retirement can apply for SSDI.

51. C: This is a requirement associated with this particular qualifying event. Coverage is allowed for up to thirty-six months in those instances where there is a loss due to death, divorce, legal separation, acquisition of Medicare, change in a child's dependent status, or other *qualifying events*.

52. B: With bundled payments, providers and healthcare facilities (separately or jointly) may receive a single payment to provide treatment for a condition. Providers usually receive payment when the treatment is completed.

53. C: A successful transition plan includes scheduling and keeping follow-up appointments, utilization of home visits, medication orders, as well as medication management that includes ongoing medication reconciliation.

54. C: Case managers who work in the home healthcare setting are provider-based case managers. In addition to home healthcare, provider-based case managers work within organizations and facilities such as IPAs, rehabilitation centers, hospitals, and behavioral-healthcare locations. Choice *A* is not a specific type of case manager, although all case managers (including those who work in home healthcare), should focus on health progression. While home healthcare case workers may provide care for patients with long-term illnesses (Choice *B*), they are not considered long-term illness case managers. Choice *D*, community-based case managers, work with nonprofit agencies as well as local state departments. Their core population consists of those communities that are low income or Medicaid and Medicare recipients.

55. A: MCOs look to reduce the risk for catastrophic outcomes; however, they have the unique opportunity to align the payer's, physician's, and patient's interests to achieve the best possible results.

Psychosocial Concepts and Support Systems

Abuse and Neglect

Abuse takes many forms and is considered the inflicting of harm on another person so as to cause distress or pain. It is typically carried out by a person who is older, more powerful, or in a position of authority over the person toward whom the abuse is directed. Abuse commonly happens within families and may be perpetrated by a partner, parent, sibling, or someone else in a relationship of trust with the victim. Populations most at risk of abuse are children, the elderly, and those with physical or mental disabilities.

Physical abuse is the easiest to define and refers to bodily harm and includes everything from hitting to unnecessary confinements. **Emotional** or **psychological abuse** is harder to define and more subtly carried out, but the effects are just as damaging as physical abuse. It involves the manipulation of an individual through guilt and shame, or by alternatively withholding and extending kindness. This type of abuse may include **verbal abuse**, which relies on insults, criticisms, shouting, humiliation, and threats. **Sexual abuse** is forced sexual contact or exposure and can include the forced observation of sex acts. Finally, an elderly or disabled person is particularly vulnerable to **financial abuse**, through the misuse, theft, or unwarranted control of their money.

It is important to recognize some of the common symptoms of abuse, as many victims will either be too afraid to report the situation or may feel a conflicted sense of loyalty to the perpetrator. A common indicator of physical abuse is unexplained (or poorly explained) bruises or abrasions and a need for frequent medical treatment/trips to the hospital. A victim of abuse may become more withdrawn, sad, angry, distracted, anxious, or aggressive. Additionally, victims of abuse may present with psychological behavioral manifestations such as bedwetting/enuresis, tearfulness, vomiting, impulsivity, acting out, bullying, and self-injurious behaviors (i.e., cutting). Signs of financial abuse may present as a sudden or gradual change in a person's financial situation and independence, evidenced by difficulty paying bills, an increased need to borrow money, and over extending on loans or credit cards.

Perpetrators of abuse are more likely to be those with a history of alcohol or substance abuse, or mental health issues. Another risk factor of abuse would be caregivers who become easily frustrated with the many needs of those in their care. Observation of caregivers is helpful for noting any concerning interactions with those dependent on them, i.e., if a person begins to display anxious or fearful behaviors in the presence of their caregiver.

While abuse is an active form of harm, **neglect** is a failure to provide care or protection. Neglect can be withholding food, money, education, protection, medical care, transportation, or any other necessities of life. The symptoms of neglect will often show themselves in a person's disheveled appearance, weight loss due to lack of food, untreated illnesses, or missed doctor visits. Neglect on the part of a caregiver may be deliberate or it may unintentionally occur in a situation where the caregiver is overwhelmed or stressed.

It is imperative that abusive situations observed by mandated reporters be communicated to the necessary authorities, whether child protective services or adult protective services. In addition, addressing the needs of the caregiver can prevent ongoing abuse and neglect. This includes education related to the needs of their dependents, anger and stress management, and effective methods of self-care. Counseling to address depression or anxiety may also be helpful.

Behavioral Change Theories and Stages

There are many different theories related to behavioral change and the stages that an individual goes through in order to achieve lasting change. The Transtheoretical Model has been successful in helping people lose weight, quit smoking, and improve their nutrition and exercise habits. While the theories of Lewin and Kotter are primarily used to achieve change in an organizational setting, they can also be applied to the individual seeking behavioral change.

Stages of Change Model (Transtheoretical Model)

The **Transtheoretical Model** is unique in that it focuses on the thinking process a person goes through even before the active process of change begins. The first stage of this model is **precontemplation**. At this stage a person is not prepared to make any change; in fact, they have not started thinking about it and may be oblivious to any need for change. In the next stage, **contemplation**, a person is still not ready to make change, but they are beginning to think about it, and intend to make changes in the foreseeable future. During the **preparation** stage, they are prepared to make changes in the immediate future and begin to actively get ready to make changes, by creating plans and setting goals. The stage of **action** is when a person makes clear and decisive changes in their life. But these changes must be sustained during the **maintenance** stage, when they become enduring habits and continue for a significant period of time. Finally, once the person has overcome both unwanted behaviors and the temptation to return to them, the stage of **termination** has been reached. **Self-efficacy**, a person's view of their own ability to accomplish something, is an important concept in the termination stage as people should now have full confidence in their ability to continue with the new behaviors.

Lewin's Change Management Model

Lewin's model of change has three distinct stages, which are called unfreeze, change, refreeze. Just as an ice cube can be melted, remolded and refrozen, this model theorizes that the same process works with people seeking change. The first stage, **unfreeze**, involves looking at a situation and recognizing the need for change. It is helping people challenge their current attitudes, habits, or behaviors, and making a persuasive case for why change is needed. During the next stage of **change**, new methods are sought, examined, and accepted. Finally, during the **refreeze** stage, these new habits and behaviors are solidified.

Kotter's 8 Step Change Model

In **Kotter's theory**, the first step is to **create urgency**: to make use of a crisis situation in order to emphasize how urgently change is needed. The next step is to **form a coalition**, that is a team of professionals and family members who will work together to support the person making a change. After that it is important to **create a vision and strategy for change**, with goals and objectives, and then **communicate the vision** to all those who are involved in the process. The next step is to identify and **remove obstacles** that might stand in the way of a person achieving the goals they set. The sixth stage in Kotter's model is to **create short-term wins** by recognizing and encouraging the small behavioral changes that are achieved. Once these small steps have been acknowledged, it is easy to **build on the change**, turning the small changes into bigger, long-lasting changes. The eighth and final step is to **anchor the change**, making the changes a permanent part of life.

The most effective means of facilitating change may be to use a combination of these theories and stages of change, depending on the needs of the individual.

Behavioral Health Concepts and Symptoms

Behavioral health includes a variety of behaviors that contribute to the health of the body, mind, and emotions. A behavioral health disorder usually refers to mental illness and substance use, but other behavior related health issues can also be included, such as smoking or obesity. Behavioral health disorders can hinder the successful treatment of medical illnesses if they are not recognized and treated. Therefore, integrated treatment of both medical and mental health conditions is the best model of care.

Substance abuse, or substance use disorder, is the persistent overuse or misuse of a substance, such as drugs or alcohol, in spite of the negative effects that it has in the person's life. Substance abuse often classifies as an **addiction**, in which the person is psychologically and physically dependent on the substance and is unable to decrease or stop taking it. Addiction includes a **tolerance** to the substance, which means that the individual has to have an ever-increasing amount in order to get the same effects, and the presence of **withdrawal** symptoms if the person stops taking the substance. Withdrawal symptoms can be physical, such as headaches and shaking, and emotional, such as anxiety and irritability. Under certain circumstances the withdrawal symptoms can be dangerous, so detox should happen within the context of proper medical supervision. Substance abuse and addiction are incredibly destructive and inevitably lead to health complications, family difficulties, and legal issues.

There are many observable signs of substance abuse, such as red eyes or dilated pupils, agitated movements, slurred speech, confusion, inability to focus, changes in sleep or appetite, or increased anxiety or aggression. A person who struggles with an addiction is usually trying to hide this condition from those close to them; this may result in lying or secretive behaviors that can indicate to family members or others that something is wrong. If several of these symptoms are observed in a client, it is important to explore the possibility of substance use through careful and nonjudgmental questions.

The case manager can then connect the client to appropriate treatment services and provide support throughout the process of recovery. The first step may be detox and inpatient treatment, followed by outpatient care. Individual psychotherapy can also be helpful and cognitive behavioral therapy has proved the most effective form of therapy. Joining Alcoholics Anonymous or Narcotics Anonymous can also assist a person in remaining clean and sober. It is important to make sure that a client also involves family members and friends in the process of overcoming an addiction, as they can help to ensure that the environment the person lives in is conducive to recovery.

Often when a person struggles with substance abuse or addiction, they may also have a mental illness, such as depression, bipolar disorder, or anxiety. Either the mental illness or the substance use disorder may have existed first and can contribute to the development of the other; some mental health issues are substance induced. This condition of co-occurring disorders is referred to as a **dual diagnosis** and can make treatment particularly difficult, as each disorder has its own treatment needs. While treatment for both conditions can happen simultaneously, it will be difficult to adequately address the mental health issue until a person has stopped taking drugs or drinking, so this would be the most immediate treatment need.

Client Activation and Readiness to Change

Client activation, similar to the more commonly used term "patient activation," refers to how involved clients are in their own treatment and how capable they are of participating in meeting their own health and mental health needs. Client/patient activation encompasses the skills, knowledge, and motivation people have to manage their own health or mental health. Clients with higher levels of activation are likely to have better treatment outcomes, so both evaluation and improvement of activation levels are important. Activation can include a client's initiating or maintaining healthy habits, pursuing available resources, or engaging in education to gain applicable knowledge. Client activation has little to do with the specific diagnosis or needs but has more to do with the client's perspective and involvement, no matter what the problem may be. Some clients with low activation may be completely unaware of their need to participate in their own treatment, while others may have the desire but lack the skills or knowledge.

Those with high levels of activation are better able to advocate for themselves with doctors, therapists, case managers, and other service providers. They also have more success in establishing and maintaining healthy, positive habits at home that will contribute to an improvement in their overall well-being. Highly activated clients will be better at following treatment advice and better at maintaining good health and mental health even when not in treatment. High activation levels are correlated with better treatment outcomes and lower overall treatment costs. Those with low activation levels, on the other hand, lack either the skills or the confidence to be involved in their own health treatment and will play a minimal role.

Because client activation levels are changeable—not fixed—service providers should do all they can to increase a client's activation level. A client can go from being completely uninvolved to taking an active role in treatment and care. There are several methods for increasing client activation. One important strategy is to assist the client in developing new knowledge and skills. This could include training in decision making and problem solving. Even teaching a client how to ask questions related to their own needs and treatment is significant, as well as providing education around their specific needs.

In addition to providing specific skills and knowledge, clients need help growing in confidence. Encouraging them to take initiative in their services and collaborating with them, instead of making decisions for them, are important means of achieving this. Another helpful strategy is to tailor support to the client's activation level. For example, clients with lower activation levels may need to take smaller steps and work on smaller challenges. Those who already have high activation levels may be able to handle bigger challenges. Those with lower levels of activation are more in need of resources to help them in increasing their levels of activation, but they are less likely to make use of such resources. Rather than providing services that low-activated clients will not participate in, it makes more sense to meet them on their level.

Client Empowerment

Client empowerment is built on the premise that a client's strengths should play an important role in the treatment. While social work and case management have historically focused on needs or problems, the strengths-based perspective focuses on the client's positive characteristics, such as their skills, knowledge, values, and other internal resources. **Empowerment** means allowing and helping the client to take control of their own treatment, and effectively utilizing strengths and skills instead of being overwhelmed by problems or deficits. Rather than focusing on what is broken or what is not working in a client's life, empowerment focuses on what is good, hopeful, and strong. Thus, instead of feeling powerless and unable to change anything in their life, a client feels motivated and inspired to make the necessary changes.

With the goal of empowering clients, case managers and social workers should not focus on client weaknesses or dictate to a client how to act. Rather, the goal is to support clients in setting and achieving their own goals, through collaboration with the case manager. Clients should be encouraged to take charge of their lives, their mental and physical health, and their future. It is the client who takes the directive role, not the case manager. The client's **self-determination**, or the freedom to choose what is best for him or her, should be recognized and encouraged. The client's beliefs and value system should be validated and honored in the decisions that are made. It is not the job of the case manager to decide what is best for the client, but rather to allow them to choose the best option for themselves.

Instead of viewing the client as a barrier to change and goal setting, the client should be viewed as the most important resource and a collaborator in the process. Empowerment communicates that it is the client who has the power to change. Often a person will fulfill the expectations someone else has set for them. For example, when it is communicated to a client that they are powerless and helpless, they will often act accordingly. On the other hand, if it is communicated that they have the strength within themselves to change, they are more likely to be empowered to make those changes. Empowerment leads to independence and helps clients gain skills they can use even when they may not have a case manager alongside them.

Client Engagement

Client engagement, the initial stage of treatment, refers to the client choosing to participate in services and actively becoming involved in treatment. There are many things that contribute to effective client engagement, but it primarily depends on a successfully established therapeutic relationship with the clinician, social worker, or case manager.

At the outset, clients may be unsure about treatment, anxious about the change process, and hesitant about establishing a relationship of trust with the case manager. The first step in client engagement is to **establish rapport**, helping the client feel comfortable and relaxed in the new relationship. Without establishing rapport, the next stages of treatment will be much more difficult. Building rapport is done through **active listening**, in which the case manager reflects what the client is saying back to them so that they feel heard. It also means using appropriate body language and nonverbal communication, such as eye contact and leaning toward the person. Other important aspects of building rapport are **empathy** and genuine care. Empathy means identifying with the feelings of the client, even if the case manager has not experienced their exact situation. A client must feel accepted and validated, no matter what information they disclose; this is what Carl Rogers called **unconditional positive regard**. All of these things will contribute to establishing rapport, the first step in building a trusting relationship between client and case manager.

Maintaining confidentiality within this relationship is also crucial to establishing trust. **Confidentiality** is the assurance that whatever the client says will not be disclosed without their permission. At the same time, it is important that the limits of confidentiality are explained to the client, and the case manager's ethical obligations of disclosure are clarified. Another ethical issue relates to self-disclosure. While limited forms of self-disclosure on the part of the case manager may be helpful, it must be done with great caution and wisdom. Inappropriate self-disclosure by a case manager or clinician can be harmful to the relationship, as it takes attention away from the client and creates confusion about the boundaries of the professional relationship.

The next steps in client engagement are to begin the assessment and evaluation, identify appropriate services, and set goals. Asking good questions is imperative during this stage, but all questions should be asked in a nonjudgmental way, ensuring that clients feel comfortable revealing personal information about themselves. When the needs of the client are fully understood and appropriate services identified, they will feel confidence in the skill and knowledge of the case manager. This will contribute to successful client engagement in services. Setting goals for treatment should be a joint effort between the client and case manager, and the client's empowerment and self-determination should be the guiding forces during the process.

There may be some significant barriers to engagement, especially if the client is involuntarily involved in services or has had a history of negative experience with other providers. Under such circumstances, it may take more time and effort to establish a supportive, positive, helping relationship with the client. In these cases, it is even more important to be diligent and patient in building rapport and trust.

Client Self-Care Management

Client self-care management is the practical outworking of the principles of client activation and client empowerment. For clients who have long-term physical or mental illnesses, it is important for them to be very involved in managing their own care. This includes both decision making related to treatment and engaging in health promoting behaviors on a day-to-day basis. For physical and mental illness, proper exercise and nutrition can significantly contribute to the management of symptoms and must be maintained daily by clients. Other management challenges can be taking medications consistently, scheduling and attending doctor appointments, and even handling changing emotions.

The role of the case manager is to support the client in self-care management. Similar to client activation, promoting client self-care management involves education, confidence building, and skill development. This must include a focus on **self-directed care**, which is informed and controlled by the wishes, priorities, and values of the client. In other words, if there is a need for lifestyle change, the client should be the one to decide what the change will be and how it can best be carried out. It is more likely that these changes will endure if a client has been the one to decide on the appropriate strategies. Another significant aspect of self-care management is **self-advocacy**, in which clients learn to ask questions and advocate for their own perceived needs. Self-advocacy is important when working with many different services providers, such as doctors, case managers, therapists, and other clinicians. Self-advocacy can also involve identifying and accessing community resources.

Informed decision making is also a critical element of client self-care management. Instead of dismissing the client as uninformed, the best method for the case manager is to help the client grow in understanding their own needs so that they can make decisions in an informed way. Clients should have all treatment options explained fully, as well as the ramifications of each. When it comes time for decisions related to health care, case managers should engage in **shared decision making** in collaboration with the client. Finally, to ensure informed and effective self-care management, clients will need **health education**, particularly as it relates to their own physical, emotional, and psychological health.

The more that clients are able to manage their symptoms and health needs at home, the less emergency and professional care they will need. Although professional help can be sought when symptoms are exacerbated or crisis situations arise, daily self-managed care will minimize these more extreme problems and help the client to enjoy better overall health and stability.

Community Resources

There is a wide range of **community resources** available, making it confusing for some clients to navigate the system and identify what would be most helpful for them. Therefore, a case manager plays a critical role in helping the client to find and utilize the community resources that would be most beneficial. When seeking resources, it is useful to look at the different domains of life—physical, psychological, emotional, spiritual, and educational—and then compile a collection of resources that may be useful for the client in each of these domains.

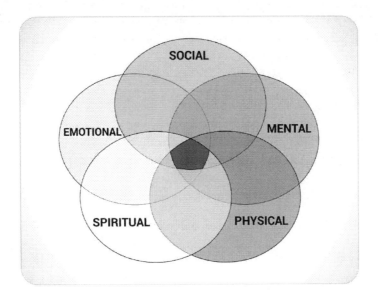

Physical needs can include food, shelter, clothing, or medical care, and there are many government programs available for these needs, such as free health care, affordable housing, and food stamps. For the elderly or disabled, their greatest need may be related to the accessibility of physical resources. In that case, the delivery of meals through Meals on Wheels or transportation services may be the most appropriate recommendation. Another help would be prescription assistance programs offered by some pharmaceutical companies to those with low income, which provide medications for free or at reduced cost. Other resources for the elderly can be accessed through the Administration on Aging and other local departments for elder care.

Ensuring the provision of adequate **emotional** and **psychological services** would first involve making sure the client is receiving emotional support from family and friends or getting involved in support groups with others who have similar struggles. For the elderly, there may be community centers with programs to help seniors connect with each other and stay active. When it comes to finding the right psychological resources, both therapeutic and psychiatric, there are many options, so the client must be involved in the process of deciding what type and format of therapy would be best.

An often-overlooked area of whole-person care is the **spiritual needs** of the client. In addition to providing spiritual support, religious organizations are often nonprofits that can assist the client in physical or emotional ways as well. Fraternal organizations may provide similar benefits to a person, offering emotional, social, and spiritual components.

Educational resources should not be disregarded, especially in the case of someone who has **mental health** needs. Whether formal training or informal learning through the library or online, there are many resources for gaining knowledge in almost any area. As discussed, education related to the individual's specific health needs is a crucial element of self-management care, client activation, and empowerment.

Calling United Way's helpline at 211, checking the U.S. government website, or conducting an internet search are easy and effective means of identifying the relevant community resources in the client's locality. Collaborating with other service providers can also make use of those who already know the client and can also prevent overlap in the provision of services. Finally, and perhaps most important, help the client to find resources through the people and organizations with whom they are already connected, as this will help their **social needs**. Not only does this encourage self-determination and empowerment by helping the client see how many resources they already have in their life, but many clients will be most comfortable with places and people they already know.

Conflict Resolution Strategies

Conflict occurs whenever there is a disagreement between two or more people or groups of people. **Conflict resolution** is the effort to find a peaceful way of solving the conflict, one that will be acceptable to all parties. In the case management context, conflict can occur when there is a disagreement around provision of services or the direction of treatment. This conflict could be between service providers and the client or between the client and family members.

There are a few things for the case manager to keep in mind when engaged in a conflict or attempting to resolve conflict among others. First, treat everyone involved with respect and empathy. Second, listen well. Actively listen to people on both sides of the conflict; in other words, collect all the facts before making a judgment. Next, focus on the problem and refrain from attacking other people and relying on emotions. Finally, make sure to keep the needs of the client as the highest priority. Once the case manager has put these principles into practice, it will lay a better foundation for exploring all possible options.

Five common types or styles of conflict resolution have been identified on the **Thomas-Kilmann Instrument (TKI)**, some being more effective than others:

1. The first is called **collaboration** and it consists of all parties working together to find a solution that satisfies everyone. This should be the end goal in resolving all important issues that cannot be compromised, especially related to the health and safety of the client. Even though this is the best-case scenario, conflict is not always resolved this easily, nor is there always enough time to devote to this process.

2. **Compromise**, or negotiation, involves everyone compromising—or giving something up—in order to also win something. Everyone wins and everyone loses. Nobody gets exactly what they want, but at least everyone gets something that they wanted. This may be the best outcome that can be expected in high conflict situations, and it may be acceptable in conflicts of little significance.

3. The third type is **accommodation**. In this case, only one of the parties achieves what they want, while the other person gives up or gives in. While this is beneficial for the person who gets what they want and can sometimes be worthwhile for the purpose of maintaining relational harmony, it will likely cause ongoing tension and conflict in the future.

4. **Competition** is a negative way to deal with conflict. This is when people take a firm stand against each other and whoever proves stronger or more powerful gets their way. In this strategy, there is little compromise or cooperation. It is important to try to find a solution by working with other people, rather than actively working against them.

5. **Avoidance** is another unhelpful way to deal with conflict, unless the issue is small or insignificant. Without bringing the issue into the open and discussing it, the problem may possibly resolve itself. More likely, the conflict will remain under the surface and will continue to grow until it becomes more difficult to deal with.

Crisis Intervention Strategies

A **crisis** can occur whenever a client is in physical danger or extreme emotional need. For example, suicidal threats or ideation qualify as a crisis situation. When a crisis arises, the very first concern is always safety. It is important to get the client into a safe situation, protected from themselves or others. After safety is established, it is then possible to assess the level of need and what should happen next in order to best assist the client.

Another important strategy is **de-escalation**. When there is a crisis, extreme emotions are usually involved. If possible, a client should be guided through relaxation techniques to help calm them down. Oftentimes, a calm and neutral party who can facilitate a conversation or listen to the client empathetically, but without feeding the emotion, will automatically de-escalate the situation. Confrontation or matching the client's emotions will escalate the situation. Allowing the client to communicate the situation fully may help them to become less emotional and more focused on the facts. At this point, the client may be able to focus on the next steps and specific tasks that need to be done. If possible, help the client to regain emotional control so that extreme options such as restraints are unnecessary.

In cases where a client is suicidal, it is important to establish if there is a suicide plan or means of committing suicide in place. These two things will determine the severity of suicidal ideation and how at-risk the client is. If it is determined that a client is at imminent risk of suicide, they should be admitted to the hospital or a mental health facility for their own protection.

Creating **crisis plans** ahead of time, in collaboration with clients, may assist them in preventing crisis situations or more quickly regaining control when the crisis arises. If clients have been part of the planning process, they may feel empowered, even when their emotions are overwhelming them. Part of the plan should be to identify the potential triggers or warning signs and have immediate steps that can be taken to avoid a crisis. This could be engaging in relaxation strategies, or calling a supportive friend, family member, or clinician.

Client Support System Dynamics

When providing services for a client, it is important to maintain a family systems perspective. In meeting the needs of someone with a significant illness, the dynamics of the family, both positive and negative, must be taken into consideration. For example, consider the role that the client has, or has had, in the family, as well as how that role may change with the progression of the illness. Every family has a system, with its own rules, expectations, and accepted ways of doing things. Family members include partners or spouses, siblings, children, or other extended family members.

Families can have a very positive effect on a client and can be the means of their best support. Adaptive and healthy families will share responsibility for financial, emotional, and physical support on a daily basis, and a family member may even play the role of caregiver. During crisis situations the healthy family will adapt and adjust, being able to meet the needs of the patient while continuing to function in a healthy way. Family members can be a huge asset to treatment, and whenever possible and appropriate, they can collaborate with the treatment plans. On the other hand, families can sometimes also prove to be a hindrance to treatment or have a detrimental effect on the client. In these cases, it is important to respect the needs and wishes of the client as relates to family involvement.

There are a few questions to ask when assessing the dynamics of a family. How do the family members communicate with each other? How does the family view and treat the patient receiving treatment? Are they domineering, enabling, or empowering? What expectations do family members have of each other? How do family members manage emotions during a crisis? How does the family deal with conflict? Are family members making decisions on behalf of the client because of physical or mental limitations? If so, are they honoring the wishes of the client? As information is gained related to these questions, it will be easier to understand what aspects of the family may contribute to, or stand in the way of, successful treatment. It is critically important to make sure that the family is contributing in positive ways to treatment. If there is mistreatment or abuse on the part of family members, this must be dealt with and reported, when necessary. Even if the family is positively collaborating with the client in accessing services, it is important for the case manager to protect the confidentiality and self-determination of the client.

As with the individual, it is important to focus on the strengths of the family and promote empowerment within the family. If needed, a case manager can provide communication skills training, conflict resolution, or a referral for family counseling. In addition, it is important to educate the family about the illness and symptoms of the patient, especially if one or more family members are serving as caregivers. This will give them better skills in supporting and helping the client. For those who are involved in caring for the patient, they may need psychosocial support and stress management.

Health Coaching

Health coaching, or wellness coaching, supports people in assessing personal health risks and developing positive health behaviors that lead to overall well-being. The field of health coaching is relatively new and is still growing and evolving in many ways. Coaching is done through education, collaborative goal setting, and emotional support. People from many different professional fields are now involved in health coaching, including nurses, social workers, therapists, and medical assistants. For those with chronic or mental health illnesses, this type of coaching can make all the difference in their quality of life. Coaching encompasses the idea of coming alongside a patient and helping them establish and move toward their own goals, choosing to make decisions that are healthy for them. It is about teaching them how to care for themselves.

As with the provision of all services, the first step in health coaching is to **engage** the client or patient in services by establishing a positive and comfortable relationship. After building rapport with the client, a coach can move on to assessing the client's readiness for change by using **motivational interviewing**. Instead of focusing on specific symptoms or behaviors, motivational interviewing focuses on underlying contributors to change, such as intrinsic motivation, self-efficacy, and belief in the ability to change. The purpose is to find what internally motivates the client and what barriers may be causing indecision and ambivalence about change. There are many things that may be causing the client to feel conflicted, and it is the job of the coach to explore all aspects with the client and help them remove any obstacles to change.

The next step in coaching is **goal-setting**. Setting goals is a collaborative process with the client. It is important to set an overall vision that reflects the client's long-term goal for health and wellness. Then it will be easier to set large goals, and for each of those to set smaller, measurable objectives. In this way, clients will take small, manageable steps at first, but always be moving toward the overall vision of health that has been established. When it comes to nutritional and health changes, it is often nearly impossible to make huge changes all at once, and most clients will have more success if they can first gain confidence by meeting smaller goals.

Finally, a health coach provides **ongoing coaching** and encouragement in the healthy lifestyle changes that have been made. This can include evaluation of the progress made by the client on goals and updating or adjusting goals as needed. At this stage, the coach may play a less involved but still supportive role in the client's life.

New initiatives in health coaching are now looking at group coaching as well as peer coaching. Both of these provide the benefit of connection and encouragement from others who have similar struggles and may be more cost effective. More research needs to be done into the effectiveness of these new models.

Health Literacy

Health literacy refers to a patient's ability to read and understand medical and nutritional terms. This includes words related to illnesses, parts of the body, medicines, and medical forms. If it is observed that a patient has difficulty reading or completing health forms, or relies on others to access medications, this may be a sign of limited literacy. Some simple, non-threatening questions can be asked about whether a patient picks up medications or fills out forms independently. If the answer is no, a health literacy assessment can be used to confirm a patient's level of literacy. Obviously, if a patient is unable to follow directions or understand the treatment being recommended by the doctor, this could be a hindrance to effective medical care.

There are now many options for measurement tools to assess levels of health literacy. Two of the most validated and tested tools are the **Test of Functional Health Literacy in Adults** (TOFHLA) and the **Rapid Estimate of Adult Literacy in Medicine** (REALM). TOFHLA has some short-answer comprehension questions and some numerical-calculation questions, and utilizes real materials, such as medicine labels and medical forms. It provides each patient with a categorical score of inadequate, marginal, or adequate. TOFHLA also has an abbreviated form and has been translated into Spanish and other languages. REALM focuses primarily on word recognition and reading grade level, not on comprehension. A patient is given a list of words and asked to read the ones that are familiar. Whichever words are skipped or mispronounced are not scored. REALM also has a shortened version, the REALM-R, which takes only two minutes to administer. As of yet, the REALM has not been successfully translated into other languages.

The **Newest Vital Sign** (NVS), which also is available in Spanish, is a straightforward test that uses a sample nutritional label from an ice cream carton and the test administrator asks a few simple questions about it to assess the patient's level of literacy. A score of 4-6 indicates adequate literacy; a score of less than 4 could indicate limited literacy.

The **eHealth Literacy Scale** (eHEALS) assesses a person's ability to access and understand electronic or internet related health resources and services. This is an important measure as e-health, the use of digital records and resources in medical care, continues to grow in popularity. Some other measurements are the **Short Assessment of Health Literacy** (SAHL), in both Spanish and English, and the **Health Literacy Skills Instrument** (HLSI), a computer-based assessment.

Because the different health assessment tools are slightly different in focus, though there is high correlation between them, it may be helpful to administer more than one assessment tool in order to attain the best understanding of the patient's literacy level. REALM and NVS are quick and easy and may be a good starting place. TOFHLA is more extensive and time consuming, and so would be appropriate in situations where limited literacy is suspected. In these cases, a more in-depth assessment would help to direct health education.

Interpersonal Communication

Interpersonal communication is the process by which people exchange ideas, meanings, and feelings with each other. It happens between two or more people and most usually refers to face-to-face communication through words and nonverbal cues, though phone calls, emails and now text messages are also important means of communication. It is very important for case managers to have strong interpersonal communication skills; this type of communication is the main focus of the job, and happens not only with the client, but with other service providers and family members as well.

Effective interpersonal communication can build strong relationships and is integral to establishing rapport, empowering the client, and resolving conflict, among other things. Skillful communication begins with active listening. One aspect of good listening is to use open-ended questions, which can also elicit more extensive information from the client. Good communication also involves nonverbal expression, including body position and facial expressions.

Along with active listening and helpful nonverbal cues, the actual content of the message needs to be clear. This means contextualizing what is being said for the specific client or situation and choosing the words that will most clearly deliver the message. Education level and cultural background are just two things that should be considered when choosing what to say and how to say it. The best way to determine if the information is being understood and accepted is to observe the reaction and attention of the listener. For example, if a client non verbally expresses anger or confusion about what is being said, it may be appropriate to stop and ask the client to share their feelings.

Being aware of barriers to communication can prevent a breakdown in the delivery of the message. Disruptive noise, for example, can distort or hide the message that is being communicated. This can include external sounds from the environment, or the way the person is communicating, through difficult words or in an inappropriate way. The barriers may also be on the part of the listener, if they are distracted or too emotionally upset to accept what is being said. Or there may be cultural or language barriers. In these cases, whatever is causing the distraction should first be addressed and the attention of the listener regained.

Effective interpersonal communication within a group can be more complex, as there are many people who have different ideas to share and different ways of communicating. A group can have a positive influence, as it takes the ideas and strengths of many people and puts them together to create a stronger whole. On the other hand, group dynamics can also suppress the voice of the individual. In groups it is even more important to make sure that people are being listened to, that respect is shown for all opinions, and that each person is given the time and confidence to share their thoughts. Each group needs positive rules and expectations that are stated clearly, and harmful communication should not be tolerated.

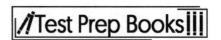

Interview Techniques

The main goal of interviewing a client is to gather the necessary information for a collaborative treatment plan. Proper interviewing can also serve to establish rapport and assist the client in developing an empowered view of themselves and the situation. While interviewing clients, it is helpful to also keep in mind the principles of good interpersonal communication, as these all apply during the interview process.

The first thing to consider when holding an initial interview with a client is the environment. The interview should be in a place, and at a time, that is conducive to the needs of the client. For example, if a client struggles with agoraphobia, the best place to meet may be in their home rather than in an office. Prior to the interview, the client should be informed of what to expect in order to decrease any anxiety that he/she may be experiencing. During the interview, very personal and potentially difficult information will be gathered from the client, so it is imperative that the client feels comfortable sharing this private information. Providing options of places and times to meet for the interview will immediately give the client some control and empowerment in the treatment process.

Another key to successful interviewing is asking the necessary questions in such a way that the client feels comfortable and relaxed in the relationship. This helps to establish rapport, which is the foundation of positive treatment and care. The case manager should clearly introduce themselves and be as honest as possible without compromising on professionalism. Building rapport can also involve finding common ground, communicating genuine care for the client, and using humor or non-threatening questions to help break the ice.

There are two types of questions that can be used when interviewing: **close-ended** and **open-ended** questions. Both are important, depending on what kind of information is being gathered. When gathering simple demographic information, the case manager may want to use close-ended questions to get straightforward answers (such as the age of the client). Using only close-ended questions will not provide the client with an opportunity to share other information that is important to them. Their struggles, fears, concerns, and needs will better be explored and understood by asking open-ended questions. Clients may not be able to easily say everything they want to, or even know exactly what they want to say. In this case, good questions can help them in the process of expressing their own thoughts and feelings. Using clarifying questions can also ensure that the case manager really understands what the client is communicating. One example of this could be, "Would you explain what you mean by _____?"

Asking questions is not the only aspect of interviewing. Interviewing also involves active listening and empathetic responding. While a client is answering questions and telling their story, the case manager should still be fully engaged. This happens through non-verbal responses and eye contact, as well as reflecting what the client says back to them. An effective way of doing this is to say, "What I hear you saying is _____ - is that correct?" The first interview will either make a positive or negative impression on the client and will influence their decision to engage in treatment.

The final step in the interview is to collaborate and agree on follow-up steps. Whether this is to decide on goals for care or when a follow-up interview can take place, the decisions need to be made with the client.

Multicultural, Spiritual, and Religious Factors That May Affect the Client's Health Status

Multiculturalism is an integral aspect of culture in the United States, which comprises people from many countries and cultures, often speaking different languages. When it comes to case management, each client will come from a different cultural and religious background. This can lead to many challenges, such as language barriers, or more subtle but complex differences. Both the client and the case manager will have their own cultural and religious biases and beliefs that will influence the way they look at treatment.

One aspect of multiculturalism is that cultures can be individualistic or collectivist, which will play a part in how the client views health and healthcare. In **individualistic** societies, decisions are made by the individual and things like privacy and independence are valued. On the other hand, in a **collectivist** society, decisions related to health may be a community responsibility, and the assumption will be that the whole family will be involved in a client's treatment. This may not only involve the family but also the spiritual or religious community as well. While upholding ethical guidelines around confidentiality and privacy, a case manager must also respect the culture that the client comes from and involve the community as much or as little as the client desires.

There are many things that are affected by spiritual, religious, and cultural beliefs. First, it is beneficial to describe the difference between spirituality and religion. **Spirituality** is a client's belief in the operation of a higher self and/or higher components of the universe. A spiritual client may not profess a certain religion but may engage in practices such as yoga or meditation. On the other hand, **religion** is a profession of belief in a God(s) or divine being and a belief in a higher order that controls the universe. Religious clients often identify by the title of the doctrine they subscribed to.

Consequently, it is important for the case manager to be aware of differing practices such as cupping, candling, acupuncture, refusal to accept blood transfusions, and dietary restrictions that could be confused with abuse or neglect when compared against traditional Western American culture. Traditional medicines of the client's culture or medical practices of that culture may be preferred over what doctors recommend. Moreover, there are gender roles that may affect the nature of the relationship with the client and the services provided. For example, there may be a gender preference with a doctor, or the client may opt out of medical care altogether when in the presence of an opposite-sex provider. Different cultures also have different views of doctors: some are held in such high esteem that they will never be questioned, even if a client is confused or in disagreement. In addition, the client's view of death and what happens after death may play a large role in decisions that are made and will be particularly significant in palliative and hospice care.

While many doctors and case managers may avoid discussing spiritual beliefs with clients, it is one of the many aspects of whole-person care that affects a client's health and cannot be ignored. The spiritual and religious beliefs of clients should not be minimized or overlooked, even when they are viewed by physicians as prohibiting or interfering with treatment. If these beliefs are important to the client, they should be acknowledged by the case manager even as education and information continues to be provided regarding the objectionable treatment. Case managers must affirm the spiritually-guided health care decisions made by the client whenever possible.

A client's spirituality, just like their cultural background, will affect all aspects of health care including views of illness and treatment. Clients may have various ideas about the causes of illness. There may also be differing ideas about the best methods of treatment, or some treatments may conflict with the

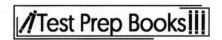

client's religious beliefs. For example, a diet suggested by a doctor may contain items that are contrary to what a client eats according to their religion. Spiritual beliefs about life and death will also play a role in decisions made by the client related to end-of-life care. As clients face the end of their lives, spirituality may become even more important to them as they reflect on the meaning of life.

In general, spirituality has been shown to have a positive impact on illness. Clients with strong spirituality may experience increased health benefits such as decreased stress and greater longevity. Moreover, spirituality tends to provide greater peace and joy even in the midst of challenging circumstances because it can bring meaning to suffering. The spiritual community that a client is a part of can also prove to be a strong social, emotional, and even financial support for the client.

Being culturally competent is a necessity for every case manager. **Cultural competency** refers to the ability to understand, accept, and respect a client's culture and religion, while recognizing one's own cultural and religious biases. Case managers cannot assume that every client will share the same cultural and ideological beliefs but must view every single client as different and coming from a unique cultural background. One obvious aspect of cultural competence is to ensure that there are no language or communication barriers, and if needed, that a translator or another case manager is available. It is also important for the case manager to understand, recognize, and support the client's specific cultural and religious beliefs. This is done by asking questions and learning everything possible about their culture. Diversity should not be feared or avoided but embraced and affirmed by the case manager. Educate and inform the client about treatment options while acknowledging and respecting their beliefs, if they are different.

Psychological and Neuropsychological Assessments

While case managers are able to conduct informal psychological assessments, it may be appropriate to refer a client for a formal psychological evaluation if there are relevant concerns. Psychological and neuropsychological assessments are conducted by psychologists or neuropsychologists. **Psychological assessments** should be done once a medical exam has been completed in order to rule out medical causes of the symptoms. The psychological evaluation is less comprehensive than a neuropsychological assessment, providing basic personality information, cognitive functioning, and psychological diagnoses. A **neuropsychological assessment** is a more in-depth evaluation of how one's brain operates. Specifically, it addresses a subject's cognitive, motor, behavioral, and linguistic functioning. Neuropsychological testing may be done when there is suspicion of a disorder linked to cognitive or neurological impairment.

Psychological evaluations are provided for a variety of reasons, i.e., employment testing, school/social difficulties in children, or people facing trials. Psychological assessments look at intellectual functionality, personality, and behaviors. There are four primary components of psychological assessment. The first component is a norm-referenced test that provides a scale of measurement to assess differences in a person's knowledge, skill, or personality. The next two components are interviews and observations, which can either be formal or informal. The final component is an informal assessment, which may be used to supplement the norm-referenced test, but with decreased scientific validity.

One tool commonly used in psychological evaluations for personality assessment is the **Minnesota Multiphasic Personality Inventory** (MMPI). There are 567 true-false questions on the test, and the results provide the client with a score on 10 scales, including hypomania and paranoia. It is an objective test that can be scored by a computer and is useful for psychiatric diagnosis. Some other personality tools sometimes used in a psychological evaluation are the **Rorschach Inkblot Test** and the **Thematic Apperception Test** (TAT), both of which utilize ambiguous images and ask the client to interpret them. These more subjective tools are based on a psychoanalytic perspective and are meant to expose a person's underlying fears, concerns, or unconscious feelings. The most popular intelligence tests are the **Wechsler Adult Intelligence Scale** (WAIS), or **Wechsler Intelligence Scale for Children** (WISC). In addition to the administration of these formal assessment tools, there is an extensive clinical interview with the client and possible interviews with others who know the client.

A neuropsychological evaluation contains many of the same components as a psychological evaluation, but in addition the neuropsychologist may test other aspects of neurology, such as memory, language, and executive functioning. Neuropsychology is intended to target things like dementia or brain injuries. When it is suspected that there is a more physiological (instead of emotional or psychological) reason for behaviors, then a neuropsychological assessment will be recommended.

The psychological assessment report is a summary of the findings from all the different assessment tools and methods. It points to themes, strengths, and needs of the client. It also provides a psychological diagnosis, according to the *Diagnostic and Statistical Manual of Mental Disorders, Fifth Edition (DSM-5)*. Previously there was a multi-axial approach to diagnosis, but the newest edition of the DSM has eliminated this aspect. The first three axes are now combined into one, providing the primary diagnosis or diagnoses. Separate notes are added to indicate any significant psychosocial or environmental factors, but these are no longer separate axes.

Psychosocial Aspects of Chronic Illness and Disability

For people struggling with a chronic illness or disability, there are many factors other than physical ones that will affect their overall functioning and well-being. A client should never be viewed as one-dimensional but should always be supported and helped from a biopsychosocial approach. Those diagnosed with a chronic illness, or those having dealt with it for a long time, may struggle with depression and feelings of hopelessness. There may also be other mental or emotional concerns such as stress, grief, anxiety, or loneliness. Some of the symptoms of mental illness may at first be confused with the symptoms of a physical illness, but it is important to distinguish between the two. Age, personality, socioeconomic status, and education level, along with many other factors, may contribute to a person's ability to adjust and cope with the new diagnosis. Conditions such as depression will directly influence a person's health and physical state, and there is a worse prognosis for those who are also struggling with mental illness in addition to a physical one.

The impact of the illness or disability will not be confined to the client alone; it will also influence the community and social structure within which the individual functions. A person who has a chronic diagnosis will play a different role in the family than previously and may need more support than they are able to provide to others. It is important to consider the adjustments a family may have to make in such situations and the different struggles they will also have to undergo in getting used to a new reality. This adjustment will be particularly profound within the immediate family and be very difficult for partners, parents, or children of the client.

While a client is receiving medical treatment for an illness, a case worker must provide whole-person care, making sure that emotional, social, and psychological needs are simultaneously being addressed. The family may also need education around the illness, and family counseling may be useful in helping everyone adjust to the changes. Identifying and connecting the client to other social supports and resources may also keep them from feeling alone and will give them others who have experienced the same things to talk to and receive encouragement from. A few other strategies to empower a client to successfully cope with a chronic illness are stress management techniques, education about the best treatments for the disease, and individual therapy. The client may also benefit from practical coaching on how to accomplish daily tasks with the limitations of the disability or illness. Antidepressants or other mental health medications may be helpful if they do not interfere with the treatment for the physical illness.

Resources for the Uninsured and Underinsured

A factor that may add to the already overwhelming and stressful nature of illness is the financial burden that faces those who are not adequately covered by insurance. While some people may have no insurance, others might have partial or inadequate insurance that covers doctor visits but not medicines or co-pays. The role of the case manager is to help the client advocate for themselves with doctors and care providers and explore options for various types of medical assistance. A case manager should also be aware of specific state and community resources that are available.

The first step is to see if an uninsured client is qualified to apply for insurance. A case manager can assist clients with the process of applying for insurance, as this can be a daunting process for many people. Insurance options can be explored through the **Health Insurance Marketplace**, run by the federal government at www.healthcare.gov, where various insurance options are presented for people in all different situations and with different levels of income. For most insurance programs a person has to apply during the open enrollment period, which is from November-January each year.

However, some insurance programs can be applied for at any point, such as **Medicaid**, for low-income families, and **Children's Health Insurance Program** (CHIP), for children in families whose income disqualifies them from getting Medicaid. **Medicare** is also available for those over 65 or with certain disabilities and can be used in conjunction with Medicaid when needed. If a client does not qualify for any of these options, private insurance may prove to be the best route for the client.

For the underinsured, there may still be higher medical costs than they can afford, often related to prescription costs, co-pays, or maxed out benefits. There are several options for getting assistance with prescription medication. Those on Medicare may qualify for additional help with prescription drug coverage through Extra Help, a program that covers the gap in coverage. There are also **patient assistance programs**, run by pharmaceutical companies, that provide affordable medications for low-income patients. Patients should ask their doctors and pharmacists for information about applying for these patient assistance programs. There are also medication assistance programs offered by individual states, some connected with Medicare and others independent of it.

Finally, there are many programs offered through nonprofit companies that connect people to free or affordable medications, disease-specific resources, or assistance with co-payments. For example, **Partnership for Prescription Assistance** connects patients to resources for the specific drug needed or to free and low-cost health clinics in the patient's area. **Patient Advocate Foundation** connects patients to a whole range of different medical-related services, including help with co-pays, and is specifically intended to assist the underinsured. Case managers should spend some time with clients exploring all the possible options for assistance with medication costs.

Supportive Care Programs

Support programs can provide important assistance to people who suffer from many different forms of illness. There are countless organizations and programs that can provide emotional, social, and financial support to clients. While some clients may have full schedules and strong support systems, additional support should at least be considered for each client. Some clients may need more help and support than the case manager and other service providers can give. Support programs should be utilized in addition to comprehensive medical care, not in place of it.

Support groups are meetings of people who have similar struggles and can share their experiences and stories with each other. They may be formal or informal, online or in person, structured or unstructured. Sometimes these groups are led by a trained therapist or clinician while other times they are peer led. Whatever the specific form they take, support groups can prevent the feelings of isolation and hopelessness that people can feel when facing a long-term illness. Popular examples of support groups are Alcoholics Anonymous and Narcotics Anonymous. There are also support groups for almost any other population or issue (i.e., parents who have lost a child, cancer, and depression). Support groups may be intended for the person diagnosed with the illness or for the caregivers and family members who also face unique needs and challenges.

There are also **disease-specific organizations** that provide help and support to those who struggle with a particular illness. For example, the **American Cancer Society**, in addition to support groups for cancer patients, also offers advocacy and education and provides practical and financial support for those with cancer. Multiple sclerosis, arthritis, heart disease, and brain injuries are just a few other examples of diseases that have whole organizations devoted to providing support to the individuals who suffer from these diseases.

Another unique form of support that may be very important for some clients is **pastoral counseling**. Qualified pastoral counselors are trained in both mental health issues and religious/spiritual issues. These counselors are uniquely able to integrate spiritual and psychological aspects of treatment and care. Many clients are concerned about their spiritual needs as well as physical and emotional needs, and pastoral counseling should be considered in these cases. Pastoral counseling may be especially important when someone is facing a terminal illness or dealing with end-of-life issues. Some pastoral counselors are certified by the American Association of Pastoral Counselors (AAPC), and this may be a good way of finding a counselor if the client is not part of a local religious congregation.

Bereavement counseling can help families or individuals cope and move forward after experiencing a loss. Whether this is losing someone to death or losing one's independence and health, bereavement counseling can help someone grieve and adjust to a loss in a healthy way. Other types of services will often end as soon as a person dies, but for the family members the process has only just begun as they begin to adjust to life without their loved one. Though grief is a natural and normal process, each person experiences it differently, so bereavement counseling should be tailored to meet the needs of the individual. Bereavement counseling may be accessed through hospice facilities or the hospital.

Wellness and Illness Prevention Programs, Concepts, and Strategies

There are many important principles for preventing illness and increasing overall health. **Wellness-focused programs** are cost effective and can contribute to a better quality of life for the patient, even those with a serious illness. The maintenance of healthy habits not only helps prevent illness but can also slow the progression of a disease. Good health depends not only on getting good medical treatment for a specific sickness, but also maintaining a healthy lifestyle and daily habits. Addressing a particular illness without emphasizing a more holistic view of health will have fewer long-term benefits.

Several basic steps should be emphasized in wellness and illness prevention programs. These are changes that everyone, with or without major illnesses, should consider implementing in their lives. The first step is eliminating unhealthy practices such as smoking, drug use, and excessive drinking. Not only do these exacerbate and cause illnesses, but they can also affect a person's mental health and relationships, which also contribute to a person's well-being. Better nutrition and exercise are also key components of wellness programs. Poor dietary habits can lead to things like heart disease and obesity, which are not only harmful but can also complicate other health issues. Daily exercise is important for everyone and can increase energy, decrease stress, prevent obesity, and contribute to better mental health.

Another important way to maintain the best health possible is to regularly and consistently attend doctor visits, and follow through with all recommended treatments, immunizations, and dietary restrictions. This includes scheduling appointments for early detection methods such as mammograms and cancer screenings. According to a person's family history of illness, there may be a greater risk for specific diseases. Doctors will be able to identify the risk factors and provide patients with particular prevention methods for these diseases.

Case managers should begin with education when encouraging their clients to begin and maintain healthy habits. Motivational interviewing should be used in helping clients to take charge of their own health and to identify any of the barriers there may be to change. It may also be appropriate to refer the client for nutritional counseling, health coaching, or addiction recovery programs. **Health coaching**, done by the case manager or someone else, may help clients find the encouragement they need to make healthy changes that will increase both the quality and length of their lives. Each client is unique, and the case manager has to be creative in utilizing different methods that will be efficient, depending on the client's level of self-determination, empowerment, and activation. For example, some clients will be self-motivated while others may need the help of a support group or weight loss program.

Social Determinants of Health

Health begins long before a patient enters a hospital and includes many factors, including social determinants of health (SDoH). Healthy People 2020 identified social determinants of health as one of the focuses of their new prevention agenda with the goal of creating environments that promote good health for everyone. Healthcare-specific social determinants of health include access to healthcare, access to primary care, and health literacy, but research has shown that economic stability, education, social context, and neighborhood environment are also social determinants that directly impact health. For example, evidence shows that patients that reside in high-poverty neighborhoods are around 25 percent more likely to have hospital readmissions.

Case managers can begin by understanding the population they serve--what are the major contributing social determinants of health (SDoH) in the specific community? By analyzing the relationships between the population that the case manager serves and the healthcare community, the case manager can begin to optimize the relationship. Case managers can explore programs in their area that address SDoH to refer patients to. Case managers in hospital settings can use an assessment to help discover the patient's SDoH that may be affecting health and discover gaps in care caused by SDoH. Case managers can bridge the gap by coordinating community resources and organizations and providing followup communication to make sure that SDoH improvements have been made.

Gender Health

Healthy People, as one of their 2020 goals, aims to improve the health, safety, and wellbeing of the LGBT community. Sexual orientation is defined as a person's attraction to another person and the affiliations that result from these attractions. Gender identity is defined as a person's sense of themselves and gender expression is the way people present their gender to others.

LGBT patients say that sexual orientation is often a factor that causes delays in healthcare, so case managers can direct patients to LGBT-friendly providers through online resources such as the Gay and Lesbian Medical Association. Healthcare providers who would like to become more educated about LGBT needs can access online resources such as the National LGBT Health Education Center. Case managers should be aware of the following factors that many people in the LGBT community face: increased risk of disease transmission, decreased lifespans, increased mental health issues with higher rates of suicide, and increased rates of drug and alcohol abuse. Case managers can help meet the needs of LGBT patients by being aware of social programs and community resources that are targeted to the LGBT community.

Practice Questions

Read the following scenario and answer questions 1 and 2.

Martha is a woman in her 50s who has recently been diagnosed with some health issues related to her poor self-care in areas of health and nutrition. She is significantly overweight, has a poor nutritional diet, and does not exercise. Martha's doctor has indicated that behavioral changes are needed in order to prevent dramatic health deterioration.

1. According to Lewin's Change Management Model, which is the first step in helping Martha achieve change?
    a. Freeze
    b. Change
    c. Unfreeze
    d. Refreeze

2. During which stage of the Stages of Change Model (Transtheoretical Model) would Martha be MOST likely to begin thinking about making changes to her nutritional habits?
    a. Precontemplation
    b. Contemplation
    c. Action
    d. Preparation

3. Which of the following is NOT a population at higher risk of experiencing abuse?
    a. Children
    b. Elderly
    c. Young adults
    d. The disabled

4. Which of the following is MOST likely to be a characteristic of a perpetrator of abuse?
    a. History of mental illness
    b. Low tolerance for loud noise
    c. Low level of education
    d. Heart condition

5. What is a *dual diagnosis*?
    a. A conflicting diagnosis from two different physicians
    b. Occurrence of a physical illness as a result of substance abuse
    c. Presence of two mental health disorders in a person
    d. Co-occurring mental health disorder and substance abuse

6. What is the MOST effective form of therapy for treating substance abuse?
    a. Cognitive behavioral therapy
    b. Psychoanalytic therapy
    c. Behavioral therapy
    d. Humanistic therapy

7. What is the BEST definition of *client activation*?
    a. Motivating clients to engage in more physical activity
    b. A client's level of involvement in the community
    c. A client's level of involvement in their own treatment
    d. A client's ability to complete activities of daily life

8. If a case manager has a client with low activation levels, what is the BEST way to increase their activation level?
    a. Provide small, manageable challenges tailored to their needs
    b. Set high expectations that will raise their level of activation
    c. Make all decisions for the client
    d. There is no effective strategy for increasing activation levels

9. What is the goal of client empowerment?
    a. To help clients become illness free
    b. To support clients in setting and achieving their own goals
    c. To set achievable goals for the client
    d. To help the client understand their own weaknesses

10. What is the first step in client engagement?
    a. Setting treatment goals
    b. Building rapport
    c. Collaborating with other service providers
    d. Interviewing family members

11. What is *confidentiality*?
    a. The case manager does not disclose any personal information to the client.
    b. The case manager makes sure that all case notes refer to the client with a false name.
    c. The case manager instructs the client to never reveal any details of treatment to anyone.
    d. The case manager never discloses information about the client without their permission.

12. Which of the following is NOT an important element of client self-care management?
    a. Self-promotion
    b. Self-advocacy
    c. Self-directed care
    d. Informed decision making

13. What is the result of effective client self-care management?
    a. Better overall health and less need for professional and emergency care
    b. Higher levels of client happiness
    c. Easier job for the case manager
    d. Decreased amount of medication needed by the client

14. Which of the following is the BEST referral option for the elderly or disabled who have difficulty leaving their homes to obtain food?
    a. Food pantries
    b. Food stamps
    c. Area Office on Aging meal delivery service
    d. A community cooking class

15. Which aspect of whole-person care is often overlooked when seeking community resources for the client?
    a. Physical
    b. Emotional/psychological
    c. Spiritual
    d. Medical

16. Which form of conflict resolution involves all parties working together to find a solution that satisfies everyone?
    a. Compromise
    b. Avoidance
    c. Competition
    d. Collaboration

17. When resolving conflict, which of these principles is important to keep in mind?
    a. Never compromise
    b. Focus on the problem instead of attacking people
    c. Avoid the people who are in conflict
    d. Speak louder to get the point across

18. In a crisis situation, what is the first and MOST important thing to do?
    a. Make sure that the client is safe
    b. Restrain the client
    c. Go to the hospital
    d. Call the police

19. If a client is suicidal, what is the MOST important information for the case manager to get?
    a. How many family members are in the area
    b. The client's food intake for the day
    c. Whether or not the client has a suicide plan or means
    d. The client's history of illness

20. What is the goal of health professionals in providing end-of-life care?
    a. To prolong the patient's life
    b. To ensure that the patient's last days of life are as painless and comfortable as possible
    c. To ensure that the patient dies in the hospital
    d. To ensure that every possible medical intervention has been fully utilized to treat the disease

21. Who should make the decision about a DNR order?
    a. The doctor
    b. A combined decision between a doctor and social workers
    c. The patient or family members
    d. Hospice care staff

22. Why is it important to have a family systems approach when providing treatment for a client?
    a. Because the client's family will likely be involved in treatment and provide significant support
    b. Because the family's wishes are more important than the client's wishes
    c. Because the client cannot make decisions about treatment without the family's approval
    d. Because doctors need the medical history of the family

23. What is the goal of motivational interviewing?
    a. To address specific symptoms or behaviors of a mental illness
    b. To convince the client to engage in medical treatment
    c. To discover the client's internal motivation and the causes of ambivalence to change
    d. To motivate the client to develop better health habits

24. In what situation would health coaching be the MOST helpful?
    a. When a person is facing the last few months of their life
    b. While a person is preparing for a marathon
    c. During pregnancy
    d. When someone has a chronic illness

25. Which of the following health literacy assessment tools have greatest validation?
    a. NVS and eHEALS
    b. SAHL and HLSI
    c. NVS and REALM-R
    d. TOFHLA and REALM

26. Which health literacy assessment tool gives the patient a list of words and asks them to read the words that are familiar?
    a. Newest Vital Sign
    b. Rapid Estimate of Adult Literacy in Medicine
    c. Health Literacy Skills Instrument
    d. Short Assessment of Health Literacy

27. Which of the following is true about interpersonal communication?
    a. It does not include phone calls and emails.
    b. It is used in personal relationships, not professional relationships.
    c. It is a very important skill for case managers to have.
    d. It consists of communication between three or more people.

28. Which of the following is an important interpersonal communication skill for the case manager to use?
    a. Assimilation
    b. Collaboration
    c. Effusion
    d. Contextualization

29. What can be a weakness of communication within a group?
    a. The room may become hot and stuffy.
    b. There will be too many good ideas to choose from.
    c. The group leader may get overwhelmed with anxiety.
    d. The group may suppress the voice of the individual.

30. What is the first thing to consider when preparing for an initial interview with the client?
    a. The treatment goals
    b. The environment of the interview
    c. The assessment forms
    d. The confidentiality agreement

31. Which option reflects the BEST use of open-ended questions in an interview?
    a. To gather demographic information about the client
    b. To explore the client's struggles, fears, and concerns
    c. To inform the client of organizational policies
    d. To assess the client's educational level

32. What's the difference between individualistic and collectivist cultures?
    a. Individualistic cultures value independence; collectivist cultures value community.
    b. Individualistic cultures tend to be poorer; collectivist cultures tend to be richer.
    c. Individualistic cultures are matriarchal; collectivist cultures are patriarchal.
    d. Individualistic cultures are not time oriented; collectivist cultures are time oriented.

33. What is *cultural competency*?
    a. The ability to quickly learn new languages
    b. The ability to handle new and different experiences in different countries
    c. The ability to explain why one's own culture is better than any other
    d. The ability to understand, accept, and respect someone else's culture

34. How is a neuropsychological evaluation different from a psychological evaluation?
    a. It takes place in the client's home instead of the office.
    b. It is more comprehensive and looks at cognitive or neurological impairment.
    c. It evaluates personality and nothing else.
    d. It requires a brief hospitalization.

35. Which of the following personality tests is commonly used in psychological evaluations?
    a. Minnesota Multiphasic Personality Inventory (MMPI)
    b. Nebraska Personality Questionnaire, Short Form (NPQ-SF)
    c. American Psychological Personality Survey (APPS)
    d. Assessment for Personality Disorders (APD)

36. What is the name of the book that contains the official diagnostic information for psychological disorders?
    a. Manual to Detect Psychological Disorders, Third Edition (MDPD-III)
    b. Diagnostic and Statistical Manual of Mental Disorders, Fifth Edition (DSM-5)
    c. Diagnosis of Mental Health and Psychological Disorders (DMHPD)
    d. American Manual of Mental Disorders, Second Edition (AMMD-II)

37. What is one of the psychosocial aspects of chronic illness?
    a. The competency of the patient's doctor
    b. Mental illness, such as anxiety or depression
    c. A client's level of involvement in recreational activities
    d. Maintenance of healthy nutritional and exercise habits

38. Besides the patient, who is MOST likely to be most affected by the patient's illness or disability?
    a. The doctor and medical team
    b. The case manager
    c. The immediate family members
    d. The patient's co-workers

39. Which government insurance program is intended to help those over 65 or with certain disabilities?
    a. Medicaid
    b. Affordable Care Act
    c. Elderly Insurance Aid
    d. Medicare

40. What is the name of the program run by pharmaceutical companies to provide affordable medications to low-income individuals?
    a. Patient prescription program
    b. Patient assistance program
    c. Patient medications assistance
    d. Patient medicine management

41. How should a case manager respond if the client's religious beliefs conflict with the recommended treatment of the doctor?
    a. Dismiss the client's spiritual beliefs and insist they comply with treatment
    b. Agree with the client's beliefs and tell them that treatment is not important
    c. Acknowledge the client's beliefs and self-determination, but continue to provide education about the treatment
    d. Refuse to work with any clients who have beliefs that are different from the case manager

42. What is a benefit a client can experience when engaging in spiritual practices?
    a. It has no noticeable or measurable impact
    b. It contributes to depression and anxiety.
    c. It makes the client more fearful and confused about life.
    d. It gives the client a more positive and hopeful outlook.

43. When should support groups be utilized?
    a. When the client feels isolated and does not have a strong support system
    b. When the client has a full and busy schedule
    c. At the beginning of treatment as a requirement for every client
    d. When the client stops attending doctor visits

44. What is unique about pastoral counselors?
    a. They only use the Bible and have no training in psychological concepts
    b. They disregard medical care and psychotherapy
    c. They are uniquely qualified to integrate spiritual and psychological aspects in their counseling
    d. They are unhelpful because they include spiritual elements in their counseling

45. What is the purpose of bereavement counseling?
    a. To force people to quickly get over their grief
    b. To minimize the loss the person is feeling
    c. To help people go through the grieving process in exactly the right stages
    d. To help a person grieve and adjust to loss in a healthy way

46. Why are illness prevention and wellness programs important for those with terminal or chronic illnesses?
    a. Maintenance of healthy habits can slow progression of a disease and improve quality of life.
    b. Engaging clients in these programs can distract them from dealing with their sickness.
    c. Patients with chronic illnesses are stronger and healthier than others so it is a good time to engage in health programs.
    d. These programs can cure terminal illnesses

47. Which of the following is an early detection method that should be encouraged by case managers to promote a patient's wellness and illness prevention?
    a. Nutritious diet and daily exercise
    b. Thinking positively about life
    c. Discontinuing any unhealthy habits like smoking
    d. Mammograms

Answer Explanations

1. C: Unfreeze is the first step of change according to Lewin's Change Management Model. The stages of change are compared to an ice cube changing shape. In order to make change, a person has to first unfreeze, recognizing the need for change and being willing to challenge the status quo.

2. B: Contemplation is when a person first becomes aware of the need for change and is willing to begin thinking about it. It comes after precontemplation, when a person is unwilling or unable to even see that there is a problem and is not thinking about change. After contemplation comes the preparation stage, when a person is more actively preparing for change and making plans. If Martha is beginning to think about making changes, she has passed the precontemplation stage and moved into the contemplation stage.

3. C: While abuse can happen at any age and to any population, the three groups most likely to experience some form of abuse are the elderly, children, and the disabled. Young adults are not considered a population at higher risk of abuse.

4. A: A history of mental illness is one of the main factors correlated with abuse. Although a low tolerance for noise or low level of education may contribute in some cases to abusive situations, neither of them is the best answer here. A heart condition is not correlated with perpetrating abuse. Other factors would be substance abuse or a tendency of a caregiver to get easily frustrated.

5. D: Dual diagnosis refers to the phenomenon of both a substance abuse disorder and a mental health disorder present in the same individual, so this would be the best response. Either one may be influenced by the other. It does not have to do with conflicting diagnoses from different physicians, nor does it refer to two mental health disorders or a physical illness resulting from substance abuse.

6. A: While other forms of individual therapy may play a part in treating substance abuse disorders, cognitive behavioral therapy (CBT) has been shown to have the most success. CBT examines a client's unhealthy or dysfunctional thought patterns as well as seeks to change the client's unhealthy behaviors.

7. C: Client activation refers to the level to which clients are involved in their own treatment and their ability to meet their own health needs. Client activation is not static: clients can increase in their levels of activation as encouraged and educated by the case manager. Client activation does not specifically refer to a client's involvement in the community, physical activity, or ability to perform activities of daily life. However, all of these things may play a role in clients being involved in their treatment.

8. A: For clients with low activation, the best strategy is to provide them with manageable challenges that meet them on their level. This encourages them as they are able to meet these challenges and motivates them to take even bigger steps. If clients are pushed beyond their current level of activation too soon, they may become discouraged by failure. It is not helpful for the case manager to make all decisions for clients, as this will serve to disempower them.

9. B: Client empowerment is when the case manager supports clients in accessing their own strengths and resources, and setting their own goals for treatment. Empowerment focuses on the client's strengths and resources, rather than problems and weaknesses. While the case manager can work in collaboration with the client, it should be the client who ultimately sets the treatment goals and decides what is best for their life.

10. B: Building rapport is the first, and one of the most significant, aspects of client engagement. The successful provision of services will be based on a positive relationship between the client and case manager. If a client does not feel comfortable with the case manager, they may decide not to engage in treatment at all. Setting goals, interviewing family members, and collaborating with other services providers may possibly be important parts of treatment, but none of these are the first step.

11. D: Confidentiality refers to a case manager's responsibility to maintain the privacy of the client and to protect all information that is shared with the case manager. Information may be shared with others collaborating in the client's treatment, but this should never be done without the client's permission. Confidentiality should always be maintained, except in cases where the case manager has received a court order. While self-disclosure on the part of the case manager is an important issue, that is not what confidentiality is referring to, nor does it have to do with what information a client chooses to share about their treatment.

12. A: Self-promotion is not a notable part of self-care management. Self-advocacy, self-directed care, and informed decision making are all important aspects of self-care management. A client should be provided with the information and encouragement to manage their own treatment and health care needs.

13. A: Effective self-care management will increase a client's overall health and will decrease the need for emergency and professional care. If a client is taking charge of their own health needs, they can become more independent and maintain better health. The primary goal is not necessarily to make the case manager's job easier or to increase the client's happiness, though these may be secondary benefits. While clients may be able to take medications themselves, unless there is a change in health status, self-care management will not necessarily decrease the amount of medication they take.

14. C: A recommendation to the Area Office on Aging for meal delivery programs would be the best option for the elderly or disabled if they are unable to leave their homes because these meals are delivered. While food pantries or other food resources may be helpful for people who have transportation, they are not the best option for this population.

15. C: While much effort is often put into accessing financial, psychological, or medical resources for a client, their spiritual needs are often overlooked. For many clients, their spirituality is an integral aspect of who they are, and spiritual or religious resources may provide a great support for them.

16. D: Collaboration is when a conflict is resolved in such a way that everyone is fully satisfied. In compromise, everyone has to give up something, in order to get something and to settle the issue. In competition, the most powerful person wins. In avoidance, the conflict is avoided altogether and not dealt with. Collaboration is the best strategy for resolving conflict, though it is not always simple or easy to solve a conflict in such a way that everyone is happy.

17. B: It is important when involved in resolving conflict to focus on the problem. A case manager should not resort to attacking people or becoming emotional. This will merely exacerbate the problem. It is also important to treat everyone with respect and engage in active listening.

18. A: In a crisis, the most important thing is safety. The first step is to ensure that the client is safe, and not a harm to themselves or others. While calling the police, going to the hospital, or restraining the client may be necessary steps to take, and may be aspects of achieving safety, they are not necessarily the first step. Safety is always the first step that needs to be achieved.

19. C: The most immediate concern is to determine if the client has a plan for suicide and the means for carrying it out. This indicates a high level of suicide risk, and thus a client may need to be hospitalized. The other answer contains either insignificant or less important information than this.

20. B: The main goal of end-of-life care is to ensure that the client's last days are as painless and comfortable as possible. Decisions around which treatments to use to prolong life are up to the patient. The main goal of end-of-life care is not to make sure the patient dies in a hospital; this should be a decision made in collaboration with the patient.

21. C: The decision about a DNR order is entirely up to the patient or family members. There should be no coercion on the part of the doctors or social workers, but they should provide information so that the patient can make an informed decision.

22. A: In most cases, the family of the client will be involved in treatment and play a supportive role for the client. In some situations, a family member may even serve as the caregiver. Whether the family dynamics are positive or negative, clients function within the context of family so it is important to understand the family as much as possible. This does not mean that the client cannot make decisions about their own treatment, or that the family's opinions are more important.

23. C: The goal of motivational interviewing is to discover and explore a client's intrinsic motivation and belief in the ability to change. It also tries to identify any barrier to change and the ambivalence a client may feel about change. Motivational interviewing does not focus on specific behaviors or symptoms, but rather on underlying causes.

24. D: When someone has a chronic illness, they may need extra coaching and support to develop and maintain healthy habits. A healthy lifestyle can slow progression of a disease, minimize the symptoms, and improve quality of life.

25. D: The Test of Functional Health Literacy in Adults (TOFHLA) and the Rapid Estimate of Adult Literacy in Medicine (REALM) are the two most validated and tested tools for health literacy assessment. TOFLA is a thorough and comprehensive test, while REALM is shorter and easier to complete.

26. B: The Rapid Estimate of Adult Literacy in Medicine (REALM) provides patients with a list of words to read. They are instructed to read the words that are familiar to them. Words that are mispronounced or not read are not scored.

27. C: Interpersonal communication is an important skill for case managers to have, as most of their work involves interpersonal communication. Interpersonal communication is the process by which people exchange ideas, meanings, thoughts, and feelings with each other. It is a part of all personal and professional relationships and is used during phone calls, emails, and in face-to-face interactions.

28. D: Contextualization is an important skill for the case manager to use when communicating with clients. There will be a barrier to interpersonal communication if the case manager is not able to use words that will be best understood by the specific client. Education and cultural background are two things to consider when communicating with different clients.

29. D: While there are many positives to group dynamics and communication, it is possible for the group to suppress the voice of the individual. Some people in a group may not feel comfortable enough to freely share their opinions and may just accept the apparent opinion of the group, leading to group think or conformity.

30. B: Even before meeting a client, the case manager should consider where the interview will take place. Depending on the needs of the client, it can take place in an office, the client's home, or another location. If the client is involved in this decision, they will immediately feel some control and empowerment in the treatment process.

31. B: One of the main purposes of using open-ended questions is to explore the client's fears, concerns, and struggles. Good open-ended questions will give the client the opportunity to share whatever they feel is important. For simple demographic information, close-ended questions may be more helpful.

32. A: Individualistic cultures tend to place more emphasis on independence, privacy, and individual decision making. Collectivist cultures place more emphasis on the community and family. Decisions are often made as a group, not by an individual. Whether a client comes from an individualistic culture or a collectivist one will probably affect how involved the client's family and community will be in the treatment process.

33. D: Cultural competency in case management is the ability to understand, accept, and respect a client's culture and religion. The case manager must also recognize their own cultural biases and understand how they may influence treatment.

34. B: Both psychological and neuropsychological evaluations examine a person's personality, intelligence, functioning, and potential psychological disorders. However, neuropsychological assessments do more in-depth assessments of everything related to cognition and the brain. If there are physiological reasons behind a client's symptoms, such as a brain injury or dementia, they may be referred for a neurological evaluation.

35. A: The Minnesota Multiphasic Personality Inventory (MMPI) is very commonly used in psychological evaluations. It is an objective test that can be scored on the computer and can help with psychiatric diagnosis. Built into the MMPI are questions to test whether someone is lying or faking answers on the assessment.

36. B: The Diagnostic and Statistical Manual of Mental Disorders, Fifth Edition (DSM-5) contains the official and current criteria for diagnosing psychological disorders. The DSM was updated to the fifth edition in 2013 and there were several changes to categorizations of disorders as well as diagnostic criteria. The multiaxial diagnostic method was also eliminated in the new edition.

37. B: There are many psychosocial aspects of chronic illness and disability, including mental health concerns, such as anxiety, depression, isolation, hopelessness, and stress. A medical illness must be viewed within the context of whole-person care and not treated in isolation. A chronic illness or disability will affect a person's social, emotional, and psychological well-being.

38. C: The ones most likely to be the most affected by a patient's chronic illness or disability are the immediate family members. One or more of the family members may even play the role of caregiver. Partners, children, parents, and siblings are the ones who will often have to deal with the day-to-day burden of care and treatment, and adjust to the patient's new or ongoing limitations.

39. D: Medicare is the government insurance program for those over 65 or people with certain disabilities. Medicare can sometimes also be used in conjunction with Medicaid to cover medical costs.

40. B: Patient assistance programs are run by pharmaceutical companies to provide affordable medications to low-income patients. Patients should ask their doctors or pharmacists about these programs. There are also other state run programs and nonprofit organizations that help with medical costs for the uninsured or underinsured.

41. C: Client's beliefs and self-determination must be affirmed and acknowledged. Ultimately, it is the client's decision about what treatments to pursue. However, the case manager can continue to provide information and education about the objectionable treatments.

42. D: Spirituality can play a very positive role in the life of someone suffering from a major illness. Some benefits of spirituality may include adding meaning to life and providing a hopeful outlook for the future. Spirituality may also decrease stress levels, prevent depression and anxiety, and lead to greater overall health.

43. A: It is not necessary for every client to join a support group, especially if they are already busy and have a strong support system. For clients who feel isolated and hopeless in their illness, it could be beneficial for them to join a support group with other people who have similar struggles.

44. C: Pastoral counselors are unique in that they combine both spiritual and psychological aspects into their counseling and are trained in both areas. For clients who are struggling spiritually, and for whom spirituality is very important, pastoral counseling may be what they need.

45. D: The grieving process after experiencing a loss is a natural process. No person experiences grief in exactly the same way as someone else, so bereavement counseling should be tailored to the needs of the individual. The goal of bereavement counseling is to help someone grieve and adjust to the loss in a healthy way.

46. A: While it may not be possible to cure chronic illnesses, illness prevention and wellness programs can help to slow progression of the disease and also improve quality of life. No matter what the sickness is, maintaining healthy habits will always contribute to overall well-being.

47. D: While engaging in a routine of being mindful and having a positive outlook on life, consuming a nutritious diet, engaging in daily exercise, and eliminating unhealthy habits all contribute to positive health and wellness, the only option listed that is considered an early detection health measure is Choice *D,* mammograms. Case workers should encourage all their patients to seek medical care. Early detection measures like cancer screenings and mammograms are part of preventative health and can potentially catch diseases before they have spread or become a severe problem.

Quality Outcomes Evaluation and Measurements

Accreditation Standards and Requirements

Many organizations look to attain an industry-recognized stamp of approval that demonstrates their ability to deliver and facilitate quality health care. There are a variety of accrediting bodies within the healthcare arena that provide validation of this ability by certifying healthcare establishments using core standards and performance measures.

Cost-Benefit Analysis

Organizations face the challenge of having to demonstrate the ability to provide quality case management services. In addition, they also must demonstrate the ability to reduce the cost of care while executing these quality case management services at the same time. **Cost-benefit analysis** enables an organization to demonstrate the value of case management activities and services. It can be difficult to prove the worth of case management services and activities due to the spending required to support and operate a case management program. There are a variety of tasks that case managers can document to demonstrate cost savings as well as case status.

Below is an example of the cost savings formula.

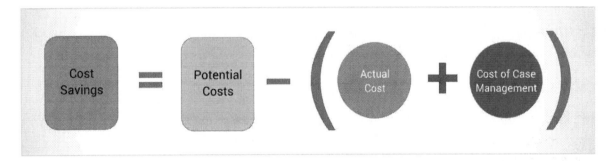

Quarterly reports should outline fees, service costs, and resources while also providing plan of care updates for those cases that remain active. Case management reports must demonstrate a movement of the patient along the continuum of care, including those interventions by the case manager that contribute to a reduction in unnecessary spending. Specific examples include hospital admission reductions, a decrease in the number of hospital days, transitions to lower levels of care, reductions in the number of emergency room visits, a decrease in medical or behavioral exacerbations, and fewer case rate negotiations. At the same time, an increase in less costly home care and outpatient services must be documented.

Case managers must create a report that tells a story in a succinct manner. Reports must present a clear picture of the patient's medical or behavioral history, treatment plan, duration of case management services, case management interventions, and outcomes. Finally, the cost-benefit analysis should provide a comparison of the costs associated with case management intervention versus the costs of managing the case without intervention.

Data Interpretation and Reporting

Case managers play a significant role in collecting data that provides an analysis of the progress of a patient in case management and provides the ability for both case managers and organizations to interpret the trends, progress, and performance measures of a case. Data and reporting assists organizations in identifying trends and establishing benchmarks for their programs.

The application or information technology system used to collect data may vary among organizations. Many software companies allow groups to customize systems to support their business needs and goals. Case managers must have a clear understanding of how to navigate these systems and document ongoing case management activities and metrics.

Business and metrics analysts leverage case management systems, and in some instances, utilization management systems, to measure utilization trends, financial costs, case management delivery, and those benchmarks for which the organization is working toward achieving. Organizations establish benchmarks internally to monitor the overall effectiveness of case management within the organization, and they also use the data to compare their performance to that of other agencies. To perform such a task, case managers must be uniform in their documentation of data and consistent with the collection of that data. Failure to follow a standardized process increases the risk for missed data or poor documentation practices. Organizations must ensure that their case managers understand the importance of accurate and consistent documentation practices.

Some states mandate that Medicaid managed care organizations provide accurate data for certain populations, such as those with special healthcare needs, demonstrating specific case management activities and measurable outcomes.

Health Care Analytics

Healthcare analytics have a significant impact on the measurement and evaluation of outcomes. Without the right tools, resources, case manager knowledge, skills, and ability, however, healthcare analytics can prove worthless in examining and measuring data and outcomes.

Health Risk Assessment

Health risk assessments (HRAs) are screening tools widely used by case management and disease management professionals to gather information about a patient's health history and current health status. These tools should be created using a team of healthcare professionals, including a physician who can provide input. HRAs enable clinicians to better understand an individual's current quality of life and care, as well as recently prescribed treatment regimens. Also, they provide some insight into the patient's current perception of their health status.

Next, HRAs provide a preliminary overview of the patient's healthcare utilization. There are occasions in which the patient's previous healthcare experience may not be readily available by way of historical documentation, and HRAs may help to uncover what are otherwise undocumented experiences, particularly for those individuals who may be more transient than others. HRAs are in use by most case management and disease management departments and are often a primary means for identifying clients who might benefit most from case and disease management services.

Health risk assessment tools vary by organization, and the method in which the data are collected and stored may also differ. The same may be true internally for the case management and disease

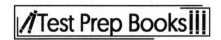

management departments within an organization for various populations and groups. The reason for this deviation between teams is a result of the need to attain, monitor, and measure different pieces of information. Some of these differences are driven by internal policies, best practices, state or federal requirements, accreditation requirements, or quality measures. There are several forms that are well known in the industry of case management and are either a component of an internal assessment or used independently to help gather information.

One example of a health risk assessment is the **Mini-Mental State Examination** (MMSE), which provides an assessment of cognitive impairment. Also known as the 30-point Folstein test, the MMSE is useful for individuals with dementia or identifying memory loss. It is not used for diagnosis but can be useful in screening for possible cognitive deficits.

Another example of a health risk assessment is the **SF-36**, which provides a measurement of the overall health status of the client and is most beneficial under a disease management model. While every organization is not using this form, there are a number of questions and characteristics that are in use by various entities. This form presents the patient's perception of their current health status and becomes an oral record of sorts that is based purely on the patient's self-report of their health history, pain, perceived limitations, mental health, social support, and environment and safety.

Health risk assessment tools can be an asset in the predictive modeling process. The HRA can support the data revealed by the model itself and can further support stratification of clients into a risk category or domain. In addition, they may reveal elements not otherwise available in a predictive model score, such as comorbid conditions that are not yet visual in the detail of claims or pharmacy data. Overall, health risk assessments should be easy to navigate and must be a component of a regular schedule.

Predictive Modeling

Predictive modeling is a tool that many organizations use to identify individuals within their population who have a diagnosis that may pose the greatest risk for preventable costs. Predictive modeling tools take claims data coupled with high-cost diagnoses to produce a score that identifies how stable an individual's condition is or is not. This results in a "risk score" that explains the likelihood that the same individual will experience a future hospitalization if there is not an episode of case management intervention and support. These tools stratify individuals within a population based on their risk over a period of time (e.g., six to twelve months).

The likelihood of hospitalization model is commonly used by managed care organizations to identify those individuals who are the best candidates for case management services over time. There are employers who also use predictive modeling data via high risk assessments to anticipate costs. This model, however, is only as good as the data available to provide an accurate picture of the patient. While it typically leverages twelve months of data to determine and handicap the model, it does mimic real-world experiences. It works best for chronic conditions including but not limited to: diabetes, congestive heart failure, chronic obstructive pulmonary disease, asthma, renal failure, and pneumonia.

Organizations target those diagnoses or conditions that are known to result in higher costs and have high readmission rates. Predictive modeling enables case management departments to establish critical interventions, implement performance measures, and develop individualized strategies to support the facilitation of specific services, in an effort to greatly reduce the risk of an unanticipated or catastrophic health event.

Predictive modeling is a proven asset to case management departments. It allows case managers to focus on those populations that will benefit most from case management intervention strategies, including outreach and education, and provides the opportunity to effectively develop a plan of care that is both collaborative and comprehensive.

Adjusted Clinical Group

Adjusted Clinical Groups System (ACG), a creation of researchers at Johns Hopkins University School of Hygiene and Public Health in Baltimore, Maryland, was developed more than twenty years ago out of a necessity to better understand the profile of a patient's morbidity and the overall presentation of some populations, allowing for the measurement of performance and quality for the purposes of capitation payment.

ACGs, formerly known as Ambulatory Care Groups, measure health status by grouping diagnoses into clinical groups using the patient's age, sex, and diagnosis over twelve months.

The ACG system has a role in assigning individuals a particular ACG value, which is in direct correlation to their anticipated or actual utilization of services.

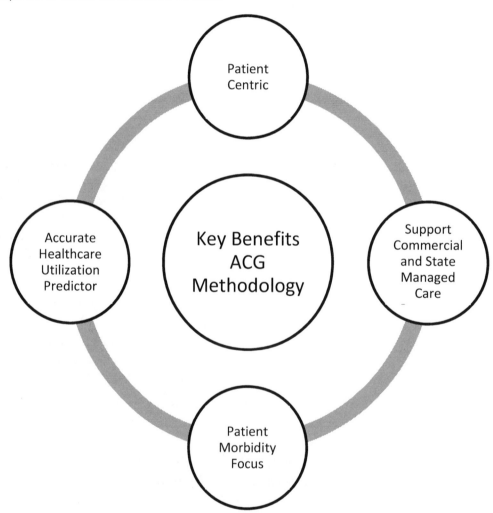

The benefits associated with adjusted clinical groups are patient centric and affect the patient and the organization. This is a model that fits the description of being patient focused, which is a key ingredient of any program seeking a way to evaluate the quality of care metrics. **Patient-centric models** tend to focus primarily on the patient as an individual, including characteristics such as their current state of health, treatment plan, and ongoing monitoring throughout the continuum of care. The focus is not only on a patient's procedures but delves deeper into a patient's morbidity.

Unlike some models that focus mainly on those populations that are complex and at risk for catastrophic outcomes, the ACG system provides for the ability to monitor both healthy populations and physically challenged persons, and it can support both commercial and Medicaid managed care programs. This system can better predict the likelihood of inpatient admissions/readmissions and emergency department visits; it can also better identify which individuals will be high cost-utilizers when compared with other models.

Use of the ACG has a direct impact on the improvement of both healthcare resource allocation and the disease profile of the population. Users of ACG should be aware of the following: There are diagnoses data (medical services and physician claims) that may need to be excluded; users must have access to the research registry and identify an index date of interest; and ACG utilizes the International Classification of Disease ICD-9/ICD-10 codes.

Over the past twenty years, the ACG system has undergone an evolution, using predictive modeling strategies, incorporating pharmacy measurements, and deploying care management applications as a component of its system. One such development has included the use of predictive modeling as part of ACGs. These models monitor future costs, potential hospitalizations, and the increased risk for increased pharmacy utilization.

Expert clinicians and the ACG system categorize ICD-9 and ICD-10 codes into one of thirty-two groups or clusters known as **Aggregated Diagnosis Groups™** (ADGs®). Patients may not be assigned any ADGs, or they may have as many as thirty-two ADGs. ADGs are assigned based on the patient's health condition. Therefore, those individuals with more than one health condition are likely to have more than one ADG. Different diseases or conditions define a single ADG. Individuals are given a unique ACG based on their ADGs. The expectation is that those who fall within the same ACG will have the same healthcare utilization experience. Both ACG and ADGs were created to better understand healthcare utilization. ADG criteria consists primarily of the severity of the illness; etiology of the illness; diagnostic certainty; specialty care interventions for the illness; and persistence of the diagnosis.

Severity of Illness	Etiology	Diagnostic Certainty

Specialty Care Interventions	Persistence of Diagnosis

The system defines ADGs as "major" or "minor." The ACG system assigns each of the medical diagnosis codes, except a few, to a patient. Several clinical and expected utilization criteria form the foundation of the ADGs. The variables include: duration of the condition; severity of the condition; diagnostic certainty (disease based on diagnostic evaluation rather than documented disease focusing on treatment services); the etiology of the condition (injury, infection); and specialty care involvement (e.g., obstetric, surgical, medical, hematology).

Program Evaluation Methods

Periodically, programs must undergo some form of evaluation to determine the effectiveness of function, delivery, and overall quality of the services provided to clients. Owners of those programs must decide if the program is addressing the needs of their customers and what opportunities exist for overall improvement. Methods used to evaluate a program include the deployment of quality management and improvement programs. There are entire departments within a company that have the role of systematically analyzing, monitoring, and suggesting ways to improve performance that will lead to the best possible outcomes for populations. Outcomes measurement provides the opportunity to examine and evaluate current practices and generate change for positive patient results. Surveys can serve as an evaluating tool that may provide insight into how well a program is operating and can present an opportunity for improvement.

Quality and Performance Improvement Concepts

Case management programs utilize a **performance improvement process** to understand better what components of their program work well and which components of their programs require modification to support the achievement of the best possible outcomes for the patient. The primary focus of **continuous quality improvement** (CQI) programs is to improve the overall quality of healthcare delivery and identify and remove potential barriers, while continuing to maintain an emphasis on both outcomes and processes of care. Enhancement of the quality of care is completed through the implementation of a specific process. Initially, the problem is clearly identified. Second, a **Corrective Action Plan** (CAP) is employed. Next, thorough observation and close monitoring of the CAP occurs, followed by a review and evaluation of outcomes. Finally, reinforcement of the required changes in processes is expected.

Case management CQI practices have been formulated to improve healthcare access and facilitation; professional case management execution and support of the client within the healthcare delivery team; client outcomes; promotion of clients' safety; and the overall improvement of customer satisfaction. **Quality improvement** examines three specific measures of improvement, including structure (physical structure and buildings), process (systems functionality), and outcome (the result). Program administrators and health providers deploy the practice of root cause analysis to identify those factors that directly contribute to mediocre performance and have a causal effect on outcomes, or those things that may lead to an adverse event.

An assortment of models may be used to measure quality improvement, and two of the most commonly seen models are Six Sigma and the PDSA Model. Both models supply a foundational framework to organizations in need of a clear strategy to measure quality improvement activities. **Six Sigma** has a primary goal of implementing a measurement-based strategy that concentrates on process improvement. It had its beginnings with Motorola during the 1980s. Six Sigma is a business strategy that boasts the ability to save millions, if not billions, of dollars. Though it began with Motorola, Six Sigma has a strong reputation in several sectors including health care. Six Sigma may use one of two sub-methodologies to achieve this improvement. The **DMAIC** (define, measure, analyze, improve, control) process is best for those existing processes that fall below specification and require an incremental improvement.

The **DMADV** (define, measure, analyze, design, verify) process assists with the development of new processes or for those processes that require more than just an incremental improvement.

The application of the concepts of Six Sigma boasts numerous advantages. Primarily, the results will include improved patient outcomes stemming from a renewed customer focused approach; problem resolution; the reduction or removal of defects; cost savings and subsequent revenue increases; and a more proactive work environment. Implementing the Six Sigma strategies also includes some disadvantages. First, it is known to create a bit of bureaucracy and foster a climate that can feel limiting. Executing Six Sigma strategies can also lead to process backlogs and limit the ability to be innovative. Nevertheless, Six Sigma is useful in healthcare and enables medical professionals to identify variances and process gaps easily in those instances where inconsistencies in performance are difficult to see.

The **PDSA model** is self-described as being a "Model for Improvement." It fast-tracks improvement within the healthcare setting and operates as a supplement to existing quality improvement models that are already in place. The model is divided into two parts: Fundamental Questions and Four Stages.

The model challenges its users to ask themselves three fundamental questions before starting. What are we trying to accomplish? Answering this question yields clear and measurable goals, which are a component in establishing what one is looking to accomplish. The answer to this question should include those issues that affect the team, leadership, and client. This effort may entail identifying industry standards, metrics, and best practices as a component of the answer. How will we know that a change is an improvement? The team will need to clearly describe how a change will indicate an improvement. This will require ongoing measurement of outcomes and show real, sustainable improvement over time. It will be necessary to collect data in order to determine if a change will truly lead to an improvement and whether or not it will be measurable. What changes can we make that will result in improvement? More than likely, the number of changes will be small in number to result in improvement, but the work to get there will require various stakeholders to achieve success.

The PDSA model involves four stages in which a process improvement plan is initiated to execute a change:

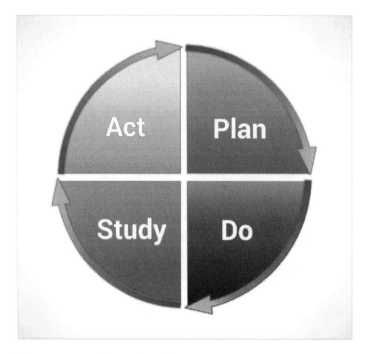

The implementation of the PDSA model involves four components.

- The **Plan phase** focuses on establishing objectives, making predictions, and creating a plan for data collection.

- The **Do phase** requires the execution of the plan (who, what, when, where) and documentation of the data.

- In the **Study phase**, the findings are analyzed and evaluated.

- The final **Act phase** involves refining the change based on the findings and planning for that change.

PDSA requires commitment and long-term planning for optimal success. This model works for pilot programs because it allows for small-scale testing before large-scale implementations. Whether choosing Six Sigma or PDSA, either model can support the facilitation of a strategy and enable organizations to demonstrate their quality improvement activities.

Quality Indicators and Applications

Quality indicators exist to enable the measurement of quality and cost of care. Organizations establish key metrics to support the process of both examining and evaluating the results of healthcare delivery by not only providers but by their internal teams, including those in the role of case manager.

Health Plan Employer Data and Information Set (HEDIS) provides insight into the ongoing effort to prevent illness. It also enables health plans to compare best practices based on overall performance. The **National Committee for Quality Assurance** (NCQA) utilizes HEDIS scores to measure the performance of managed care organizations. Certified auditors have a responsibility to validate HEDIS results, following the process instituted by NCQA.

A component of HEDIS is the CAHPS® 5.0 survey. The **CAHPS® 5.0 survey** examines the satisfaction that members do or do not have with the following areas: claims processing, customer service, and access to care.

Benchmarking is another method that allows for the analysis of healthcare delivery, trends, and best practices. **Benchmarks** are useful in that they permit the comparison of apples to apples. This is especially true when audits are internal to an organization. In addition, benchmarking also allows the comparison of results with state, regional, or national organizations that are similar in structure. For example, the average length of stay or number of bed days may be a metric that is monitored and even tied to the performance of an organization.

Industry benchmarks in managed care organizations include: acute-care admissions per thousand; acute-care bed days per thousand; skilled nursing bed days per thousand; home care admissions per thousand; and home care visits per thousand. The benchmarking exercise can also help to identify processes that have an opportunity for improvement. The exercise supports monitoring of consistency in practice while also enabling compliance with quality standards. Patients, caregivers, providers, payers, and a variety of other participants in the patient's care should be a part of evaluating their experience with the case management. Their feedback is critical in the evaluation of the overall effectiveness of a program. Also, case managers are often the face of the business, and this means that there must be a measurement of performance.

Sources of Quality Indicators

Quality indicators come from a variety of sources that are discussed in this guide, including the Centers for Medicare and Medicaid Services (CMS); the Utilization Review Accreditation Commission (URAC); the National Committee for Quality Assurance (NCQA); the National Quality Forum (NQF); and the Agency for Healthcare Research and Quality (AHRQ). **Quality indicators** are used to establish a set of standards that may be used to evaluate and measure the quality of care.

Centers for Medicare and Medicaid Services

The CMS requires providers (e.g., professionals and hospitals) to submit **clinical quality measures** (CQMs) to demonstrate their ability to provide care that is safe, effective, efficient, timely, and patient centered. CMS updates CQMs or clinical quality measures each year. CQMs provide a method of evaluation to measure and monitor the quality of care that healthcare providers and hospitals deliver. Key measurements include: cost effectiveness; safety; health outcomes; clinical processes; coordination of care and patient engagement; and adherence. Providers utilize certified Electronic Health Record (EHR) technology to submit their CQM data. EHR technology allows providers to share data about their patients while also gaining a full perspective on those trends and outcomes associated with the patient and the quality of care.

Utilization Review Accreditation Commission

URAC, formerly known as the Utilization Review Accreditation Commission, serves as a nonprofit accrediting body for healthcare organizations, enabling them to facilitate quality care. Various stakeholders are used to develop core measures and standards. URAC accreditation is an industry-recognized validation that demonstrates an excellence in quality and care coordination.

URAC's performance measures provide the opportunity for awareness as it relates to reviewing healthcare quality and opportunities for quality improvement. URAC selects performance measures that will provide value to various stakeholders, including consumers and purchasers. Also, these measures are compared with other reported measures from other entities, such as AHRQ National Measures Clearing House and NQF.

Measures must demonstrate relevance, feasibility, and appropriateness. The review process includes a close examination by URAC Measures Advisory Group and URAC Health Standards Committees, as well as other advisory committees. These committee positions are filled by clinicians, providers, consumers, and experts who specialize in these metrics. Those measures are subject to public comment. The process concludes with a final review and adoption by the URAC board of directors.

Measures are divided into the categories of mandatory measures and exploratory measures.

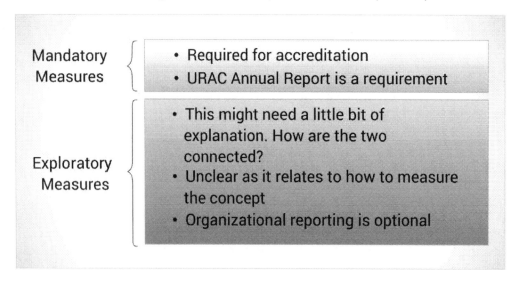

URAC incorporates various performance measures into its accreditation programs. The measures include: Disease Management; Health Plan with Health Insurance Exchange; Health Plan; Specialty Pharmacy; Mail-Service Pharmacy; Drug Therapy Management; Case Management; and Comprehensive Wellness. Organizations with URAC accreditation have a requirement to gather data that tie to the measures and report them each year to URAC by a specific date.

URAC operates a case management accreditation program with a primary focus on enabling health plans to build a program that is actively capable of managing transitions effectively, ultimately supporting the goal of reducing the risk for inpatient admissions as well as having a positive impact on health outcomes. Any organization such as an accountable care organization, hospital, managed care organization, long-term care organization, or behavioral health organization, just to name a few, may apply for URAC accreditation.

Organizations that receive the URAC accreditation can meet the performance measures and standards as set forth by this accrediting body. Case management entities now have the option of pursuing the designation for Transitions of Care. Measures included in the case management area of the URAC accreditation consists of the following domains: medical readmissions; disability and workers' compensation: percentage of those medically released to return to work; timeliness of response to complaints; consumer satisfaction; and a three-item care transition measure.

National Committee for Quality Assurance

NCQA uses HEDIS to accredit and monitor the quality of healthcare delivery activities. HEDIS consists of approximately eighty-one measures, and more than ninety percent of health plans in America use it to gauge the performance of organizations that are associated with care and service. HEDIS measures can improve health plans by identifying opportunities for improvement. HEDIS measures concentrate on health issues that affect Americans, including breast cancer screenings, comprehensive diabetes care, asthma medication use, and beta-blocker treatment following a heart attack.

Certified auditors assess the validity of HEDIS results using a NCQA-designed method. HEDIS measures form the basis of health plan report cards. The report card that is available to consumers provides ratings for: access and service; qualified providers; staying healthy; getting better; and living with illness. Organizations submit HEDIS measures via the HEDIS Data Submission System which includes the Healthcare Organization Questionnaire (HOQ) and the Interactive Data Submission System (IDSS).

NCQA works to utilize evidence-based research to improve the quality of healthcare. Accreditation through NCQA enables organizations to demonstrate that they are qualified to provide a higher standard of care and services. Also, as a result of this accreditation, organizations prove that they adhere to regulatory requirements, thus allowing them to stand out from those establishments that are not accredited. NCQA collaborates with state and government entities to create healthcare policies and are always seeking the best way to provide quality care. NCQA is the gold standard of accrediting bodies for various entities including: health plans; provider organizations; health plans contracting organizations; stand-alone vendors; managed behavioral health organizations; and community care teams.

Health plans seek accreditation from NCQA for different programs, including health plan-specific accreditation, disease management, case management, wellness and health promotion programs, and case management for long-term services and support programs. Health plans may seek NCQA accreditation to support their efforts in not only receiving market advantage but also request-for-proposal requirements.

NCQA provides a report that ranks and reports on varying health insurance companies and helps to communicate how well a managed care organization is doing in the prevention of illness. Consumers can use HEDIS to compare the performance of one health plan with another. NCQA utilizes a standard set of performance measures that defines key dimensions of care for individuals with the following conditions: asthma, diabetes, chronic obstructive pulmonary disease, heart failure, and ischemic vascular disease. Also, NCQA reviews influenza and pneumococcal vaccinations along with tobacco use as components of their performance measures framework.

Organizations may have multiple programs that receive accreditation, and they are responsible for the development and operations of these programs. Those who are unable to demonstrate the ability to meet NCQA standards will be denied. Disease management organizations who can meet some or all of the standards may receive accreditation within one of three levels.

The three levels of disease management accreditation are: Accredited, Accredited with Performance Reporting, and Provisional Accreditation. **Accredited** is the highest level of accreditation and tells the industry that an organization either meets or exceeds NCQA standards. Next, **accredited with performance reporting** is the level of accreditation for a disease management organization in which an organization is required to provide reporting of their disease management measures. While the organization did meet or exceed NCQA standards, NCQA still expects to see a report. Finally, **provisional**

accreditation alerts the industry that a disease management team does not meet all of the NCQA guidelines or standards.

However, they do have an opportunity to take action within the next twelve months to attain a higher accreditation status.

Case management accreditation requires an organization to demonstrate its ability to guarantee the safe transition of its members between various levels of care and settings. Organizations must show their capacity to not only effectively provide case management services but to also adequately coordinate care. Case management programs receive accreditation based on how their performance compares to NCQA Guidelines and Standards and may dictate the term for which they are accredited. Those organizations who fail to meet NCQA requirements during the Accreditation Survey are denied NCQA status. Agencies may be accredited for a three-year period or receive accreditation for a two-year period. A three-year accreditation is the highest level of accreditation, demonstrates a high level of performance, and is a testimony to the degree of services available.

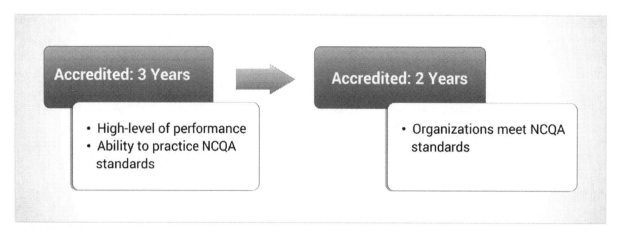

Programs that manage long-term services and supports such as health plans, independent living centers, and case management organizations, are eligible to seek NCQA accreditation for their program. Organizations that demonstrate an ability to manage transitions between levels of care or long-term services and supports (LTSS) settings, the ability to perform quality individualized assessments, and the capacity to handle critical incidents may be eligible for NCQA accreditation. As more and more managed care organizations contract to service this population, NCQA accreditation becomes that much more attractive, as it serves as a testimony to the quality of services that are available to this population and how well the organization is able to facilitate and manage those services.

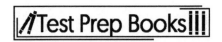

National Quality Forum

The **National Quality Forum** (NQF) mission entails the maintenance of a portfolio of performance measures. These performance measures have the endorsement from the NQF, which allows for the measurement and quantification of healthcare processes, outcomes, patient perceptions, and organizational structure and/or systems that have a direct impact on the ability to deliver high-quality care.

NQF endorses performance measures, best practices, frameworks, and reporting guidelines utilizing a Consensus Development Process (CDP). This process enables NQF to cautiously weigh the needs and interests of various stakeholder groups that represent the healthcare arena.

NQF Quality Measures

Examples of a few Composite NQF quality measures include:

- Comprehensive Diabetes Care: Hemoglobin A1c (HbA1c) Testing
- Comprehensive Diabetes Care: Hemoglobin A1c (HbA1c) Poor Control
- Comprehensive Diabetes Care: Hemoglobin A1c (HbA1c) Eye Exam Performed

Examples of Outcomes NQF quality measures include:

- Acute Stroke Mortality Rate (IQI 17)
- Asthma in Younger Adults Admission Rate
- Bacterial Pneumonia Admission Rate (PQI 11)

Examples of Structure NQF quality measures include:

- Adoption of Medication e-Prescribing
- Cultural Competency Implementation Measure
- Ability to Use Health Information Technology to Perform Care Management at the Point of Care

Examples of Process NQF quality measures include:

- Adherence to Chronic Medications
- Adherence to Statins
- Advance Care Plan
- Age-Related Macular Degeneration (AMD): Counseling on Antioxidant Supplement

NQF allows for public reporting on multiple facets of the healthcare delivery system. The NQF standards are considered to be the "gold standard" in measuring the quality of healthcare.

Hospitals, healthcare systems, and government agencies, including the Centers for Medicare and Medicaid Services, can use performance measures upon endorsement by the NQF for public reporting and quality improvement. In those instances, where a performance metric is not yet in place, a "practice" may serve as a method of providing the necessary structure to evaluate the creation, expansion, and modification of a new or existing program. A practice provides organizations with a pathway for improved outcomes.

NQF uses a set of performance-based standards that multiple groups including states, the federal government, and private sectors, recognize and utilize in the evaluation of the quality of performance and overall contribution to improving care.

NQF comprises members that represent coalitions, physicians, nurses, hospitals, ancillary agencies, and quality improvement organizations, as well as private and public entities. NQF has a board of directors that has four committees responsible for facilitating NQF activities. Those committees include: The Leadership Network; National Priorities Partnership; Health IT Advisory Committee; and Consensus Standards Approval Committee.

Each committee or group has a distinct role for the work that they perform, and leverages chosen experts to execute various tasks that enable standards to be put into place.

The Leadership Network	National Priorities Partnership	Health IT Advisory Committee	Consensus Standards Approval Committee
• Guides program convening • Directs education • Guides recognition programs	• 48 organizations • Healthcare influence	• Guides work around the health IT portfolio • Advisory role for health IT project	• Review of consensus standards • Leverage healthcare quality improvement and performance measures knowledge

NQF utilizes eight member councils to support the task of improving the quality of healthcare and building accord. The eight councils include the Consumer Council; the Health Plan Council; the Health Professionals Council; the Provider Organizations Council; the Public/Community Health Agency Council; the Purchasers Council; the Quality Measurement, Research, and Improvement Council; and the Supplier and Industry Council.

Agency for Healthcare Research and Quality

AHRQ provides the opportunity for healthcare improvement by sharing research information that improves the accessibility, effectiveness, efficiency, and quality of health care that consumers receive. For professionals, AHRQ provides access to research data, statistics, and evidenced-based best clinical practices that can have a significant impact on those decisions made by clinical professionals. Clinical guidelines can greatly support clinical professionals in their decision-making activities. They serve as a significant tool to not only reinforce clinical decisions, but they are sometimes easily accessible by both the patient and the physician.

The **National Guideline Clearinghouse™** (NGC) provides healthcare professionals access to a wide variety of clinical practice guidelines. These guidelines are public and readily accessible by both professionals and clients. Therefore, patients also have the ability to access this information and interpret the potential best treatment options and possible risks associated with their condition and treatment. The guidelines are written in a patient-friendly way, making them easy to read and understand. This area of AHRQ provides specific patient-centered outcomes that outline the most effective medical treatments for a particular condition based on current research.

The **United States Preventive Services Task Force** (USPSTF) is composed of national experts who function independently to provide evidence-based recommendations regarding those preventive services that improve the health of Americans, including healthcare screenings, preventative medications, and primary care settings. USPSTF utilizes the expertise of sixteen volunteer members who operate within various fields of primary and preventative care including: behavioral health, nursing, internal and family medicine, obstetrics, and gynecology. AHRQ has a pivotal role in supporting research initiatives in the realm of patient safety and quality improvement. This research provides insight into patient safety threats and the overall impact of medical errors. Research in this area by AHRQ includes medical liability reform, patient safety, and tools to improve performance and patient safety.

AHRQ participates in efforts to reduce **healthcare-associated infections** also known as **HAIs**. With one in twenty-five patients suffering from HAIs, AHRQ supports research initiatives that are designed to identify those methods that organizations can utilize to decrease the risk. As a result of the HAI program, new tools and resources, such as toolkits and checklists, are made available for use by organizations to aid in the task of preventing HAIs and improving patient safety in a variety of settings, including nursing homes, long-term care facilities, and acute care facilities such as hospitals and physician offices.

Core measures enable reporting of quality measures that best align to the improvement of patient outcomes. **Core measures** provide a critical pathway of evidenced-based treatments that decrease the risk for complications commonly seen in certain conditions including but not limited to the following: perinatal care, stroke, asthma in children, substance use, and heart failure. CMS publishes groups of core measures and CQMs, also known as clinical quality measures.

The **Health Information Technology for Economic and Clinical Health** (HITECH) Act, which was signed into law by President Obama in 2009 as a component of the American Recovery and Reinvest Act of 2009, was drafted to support and expedite the adoption of EHR-provided incentives to those providers who adopted the implementation and use of EHR systems through 2015. The HITECH Act increases the accessibility and exchange of **Protected Health Information** (PHI) and supports the electronic exchange of health information using EHR and EMR (Electronic Medical Record) information. Under this act, patients or their appointed designees can gain access to their PHI or medical charts in an electronic format. This access enables patients to access their complete medical history and provides an enhanced method for information sharing among providers.

Providers and organizations must report security breaches related to electronic PHI (ePHI) as soon as it occurs per established requirements or they will face civil and/or criminal penalties. Also, the HITECH Act calls for physicians and hospitals that have meaningful use attestation to perform a HIPAA (Health Insurance Portability and Accountability Act) security risk assessment. There are three stages of meaningful use. To move between stages, providers must demonstrate the ability to function within each of the stages for two years before they can proceed to the next one.

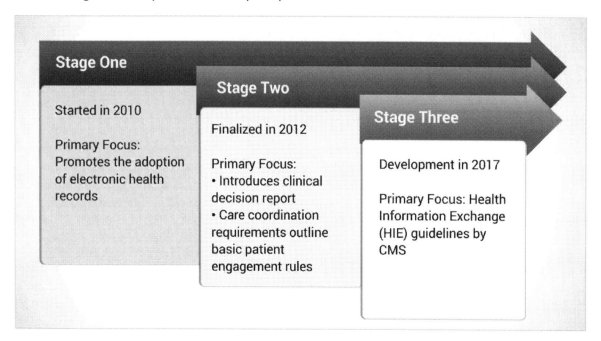

Due to a lack of budget or progress, some organizations have elected to opt-out of stage two and stage three. While HIPAA and the HITECH Act are standalone laws, they do have requirements that directly impact the other.

The Agency for Healthcare Research and Quality (AHRQ) uses Quality Indicators (QIs) to measure the quality of healthcare and may assist in the identification of quality concerns as well as identify areas of opportunity for additional research and study. AHRQ Quality Indicators are classified into four categories: Prevention QIs; Inpatient QIs; Patient Safety QIs; and Pediatric QIs.

Prevention Quality Indicators

Prevention Quality Indicators (PQIs) are population-driven with some adjustments that are tied to age and gender. PQIs can flag issues that need additional investigation. They are an inexpensive screening mechanism for opportunities to improve care. PQIs highlight access to care challenges and carefully examine community healthcare systems and outpatient services that are available and can assist in the prevention of inpatient admissions. They form the foundation for evaluating community-based programs that are in place and determining where gaps exist. PQIs also serve as a component of comparative public reporting, trending, and pay-for-performance initiatives.

Examples of PQIs include but are not limited to the following:

- PQI 01 Diabetes Short-term Complications Admission Rate
- PQI 07 Hypertension Admission Rate
- PQI 08 Heart Failure Admission Rate
- PQI 11 Bacterial Pneumonia Admission Rate
- PQI 12 Urinary Tract Infection Admission Rate

Inpatient Quality Indicators

Inpatient Quality Indicators (IQIs) assess the quality of inpatient care. This assessment is done using the data that is a component of a hospital discharge abstract or subset. Indicators that accompany this data include mortality, utilization, and volume.

Examples of IQIs include but are not limited to the following:

- IQI 16 Heart Failure Mortality Rate
- IQI 17 Acute Stroke Mortality Rate
- IQI 19 Hip Fracture Mortality Rate
- IQI 21 Cesarean Delivery Rate, Uncomplicated
- IQI 23 Laparoscopic Cholecystectomy Rate

Inpatient Quality Indicators allow hospitals to identify and target areas for study and investigation. They are representative of the quality of care that is available in a hospital and risks for excessive surgeries, high mortality, and volumes of procedures.

Patient Safety Quality Indicators

Patient Safety Quality Indicators (PSIs) provide information for events such as surgeries, procedures, and childbirth. They allow for an assessment of adverse events incidence and hospital complications. Administrative data commonly found in the discharge record provides this information. The goal of retrieving this information is to enhance the overall safety of patient care delivery.

Patient Safety Indicators provide opportunities for the following:

- Comparative public reporting
- Trending
- Pay-for-performance initiatives
- Identification of avoidable complications

Examples of Patient Safety Indicators include but are not limited to the following:

- PSI 03 Pressure Ulcer Rate
- PSI 13 Post-operative Sepsis Rate
- PSI 14 Post-operative Wound Dehiscence Rate
- PSI 26 Transfusion Reaction Rate
- PSI 27 Perioperative Hemorrhage or Hematoma Rate

Pediatric Quality Indicators

Pediatric Quality Indicators (PDIs) concentrate on potentially preventable complications and errors that affect the pediatric population. **Neonatal Quality Indicators** are also an element of the Pediatric Quality Indicators. The indicators provide a screening of problems that might have otherwise been prevented and also give insight into opportunities for risk adjustment where applicable. Area-level indicators that identify conditions that are preventable with outpatient care, as well as potential safety risks or issues that might take place during the hospital stay, are also examined.

Aspects of care that are measured by CQMs vary. Common areas of the measurement process include: health outcomes, clinical processes, patient safety, use of healthcare resources, timeliness of care coordination, frequency and quality of patient engagements, population and public health, and general adherence to clinical guidelines. Organizations must submit CQMs to receive incentives associated with the Medicare and Medicaid Electronic Health Record Incentive Program.

National Quality Strategy

The Affordable Care Act required that HHS create a strategy to improve healthcare delivery, so the Agency for Healthcare Research and Quality created the National Quality Strategy (NQS) in 2011. The National Quality Strategy begins with the "Triple Aim" developed by IHI, which is to deliver affordable care, increase patient satisfaction, and create healthier communities. To help reach these three aims, the AHRQ further included six priorities which eventually became six domains. The Six NQS Domains are: Patient Safety; Patient/Family Engagement; Care Coordination and Communication; Effective Clinical Processes, Prevention, and Treatment Practices; Promoting Public Health; and making Quality Care Affordable. CMS aligned with AHRQ to release the CMS Quality Strategy, which uses the same triple aim and six goals to describe their quality strategy.

Types of Quality Indicators

There are multiple types of quality indicators that organizations, hospitals, and professional providers may measure, including clinical, client, financial, productivity, and utilization indicators. Much of the quality indicator data is gathered through various data sources already in place.

Clinical Indicators

Case management programs may leverage a variety of clinical indicators, but they are mainly driven by the type of program in place and the population it is serving. **Clinical indicators** enable case management programs to evaluate the efficiency in which assessments, plans of care, and appropriate treatment protocol are being executed.

While accrediting bodies such as NCQA and URAC may drive certain metrics that are being tracked and managed, case management programs may then use those pre-established metrics to validate those indicators that are monitored and documented closely. This study guide has already highlighted a few examples in which a condition drives the metric. Conditions that have key indicators assigned to them include but are not limited to the following: diabetes; congestive heart failure, stroke, renal failure, HIV, acute myocardial infarction, pneumonia, and hypertension.

Financial Indicators

Financial and utilization indicators are similar if not the same. How organizations choose to use the data are what categorizes the indicator. **Financial indicators** are closely related to cost effectiveness and cost savings. Common metrics consist of a close look at average length of stay, outlier rates, readmission, emergency room diversion, and outpatient services such as home care. Case management costs and the level of skill required to support a case management model may be another metric that organizations elect to monitor. For example, the cost to hire a registered nurse or social worker to facilitate services differs from the cost of hiring a non-licensed employee to facilitate administrative duties such as entering service requests into a system.

Productivity Indicators

Organizations often track productivity to demonstrate need of services, validate staffing models, and establish client acuity. Data collection of **productivity indicators** for case managers may concentrate heavily on time, tasks, and activities. Each time a case manager completes an activity or task, they enter that information into a case management software that calculates their productivity. For example, an organization may leverage software that calculates the number of times a case manager executes a single task every day with the amount of time it takes to complete that task. The total number of hours is divided into the total hours worked to demonstrate the amount of productivity.

Organizations can collect this information to validate if case managers are as productive as they should be for a case given the acuity of a client, and the data enables leaders to extract reports that allows them to visualize the overall productivity of not only the case manager, but departments as well.

Utilization Indicators

Utilization indicators are tracked to not only evaluate the effectiveness of case and disease management programs but general trends and behaviors of the population that is being served. Utilization indicators that are measured to evaluate the overall effectiveness of a program for clients may include an evaluation of multiple elements that include: encounters data that provides month-to-date and year-to-date encounters information by product line for both ambulatory and inpatient services; average length of stay, which provides a comparison of benchmark length of stay detail to that of a facility; emergency department visits; readmissions within 30 days; daily census reporting, which provides an overview of budgeted inpatient days per 1000 to current inpatient days per 1000 with a seven- and thirty-day trend; acute care utilization (e.g., hospitalizations); outpatient services utilization (e.g., home care); and time to access (e.g., potential delays in care). Other indicators under review could include an evaluation of how departments utilize their case management staffing models to support client and provider needs.

Client Experience Indicators

The collection of **client experience indicator** data is pulled from data that is the result of information provided by the client. Data collection may come from surveys or may also be the result of random case reviews. Common dimensions or indicators of the customer's experience are frequently concerning service and providers. While there are a number of subsets that also tie into these two areas such as access, efficiency (timeliness), and engagement by the business owners of various events, most surveys or evaluations will focus on these two items. They examine things such as treatment, communication with professionals, and responsiveness, as well as trustworthiness and cultural sensitivity. Each of these indicators has a significant impact on the client experience and are taken seriously by accrediting bodies.

Evidence-Based Care Guidelines Related to Case Management

Case managers are constantly being tasked with making sure patients are being given high-quality care in a cost-effective way, and to do so efficiently, evidence-based care guidelines should be used. Evidence-based guidelines for common illnesses can help point case managers and teams to where a patient should transition to next, and what resources could be most effective for the patient. Case managers should stay up-to-date on case studies that impact their area of work and use scientific evidence to back up practice. For example, if a new study shows decreased readmission rates when home health and telehealth are used for two weeks post discharge, the case manager must bring this information to their hospital and advocate for this to be the new discharge plan. Avoiding reimbursement penalties for readmission rates may offset the cost of these additional services.

Practice Questions

1. Which of the following is an accurate statement about the Case Load Capacity Calculator?
   a. The Case Load Capacity Calculator may be purchased on a sliding scale fee.
   b. The Case Load Capacity Calculator may be purchased for a fixed price.
   c. The Case Load Capacity Calculator is free to those seeking to use it.
   d. The Case Load Capacity Calculator is free to government agencies only.

2. What are the four categories of the Caseload Matrix?
   a. Initial elements impacting caseload, comprehensive needs assessment impacting caseload, case management interventions, and outcomes
   b. Case management elements impacting caseload, case management needs assessment impacting caseload, case management interventions, and outcomes
   c. Quality elements impacting caseload, standardized needs assessment impacting caseload, case management interventions, and outcomes
   d. Primary elements impacting caseload, general needs assessment Impacting caseload, case management interventions, and outcomes

3. Which term describes the practice of organizations looking to demonstrate the value of case management activities and services?
   a. Cost-effective comparison
   b. Health benefit ratio
   c. Medical cost ratio
   d. Cost-benefit analysis

4. Which of the following tools is an example of an industry-recognized health risk assessment?
   a. Case Mix Assessment Tool
   b. Mini-Mental State Examination
   c. Six Sigma
   d. PDSA

5. What is the practice that is commonly used by organizations to identify those people within their population who pose the greatest risk for preventable costs?
   a. Predictive guidelines
   b. Predictive forecasting
   c. Predictive analysis
   d. Predictive modeling

6. What is the average number of months used by most predictive models to review data?
   a. 6
   b. 9
   c. 12
   d. 18

7. Which of the following groups were developed out of the necessity to better understand the profile of a patient's morbidity and the overall presentation of populations?
   a. Adjusted Clinical Groups
   b. Quality Indicator Groups
   c. Modified Indicator Groups
   d. None of these

8. Which programs improve the overall quality of healthcare delivery?
   a. Collaborative Quality Indicator Management Programs
   b. Continuous Quality Improvement (CQI) Programs
   c. The Agency for Quality Improvement
   d. Provisional Quality Improvement Programs

9. What practice enables organizations to monitor trends and compare "apples to apples" in their evaluation of performance and achievement of metrics?
   a. Benchmarking
   b. Metric calculation
   c. Trending management
   d. Performance management

10. Which organization operates a case management accreditation program?
   a. URAC
   b. AHRQ
   c. NQAURP
   d. NQF

11. Which agency compares its measures with other reported measures from other entities, such as AHRQ National Measures Clearing House and NQF?
   a. NCQA
   b. URAC
   c. Quality Measures Coalition
   d. National Transitions of Care Coalition

12. What action is taken by NQCA for organizations that fail to meet NCQA requirements during the Accreditation Survey?
   a. They are initially provided with a probationary NCQA status
   b. They are granted temporary NCQA status for a six-month period
   c. They are denied NCQA status
   d. They are provided a 14-day window to make changes

13. Which of the following is a level of disease management NCQA accreditation?
   a. Accredited with Qualifying Credentials
   b. Accredited with Performance Rating Standard
   c. Provisional Accreditation
   d. Accreditation with Provisional Guidelines

14. What NCQA data enables consumers to compare one health plan with another?
    a. HEDIS
    b. National Clearinghouse Guidelines Reporting
    c. URAC reporting
    d. Predictive modeling data

15. Which of the following is the period of time for which an organization may receive accreditation by NCQA?
    a. One year
    b. Two years
    c. Four years
    d. Five years

16. What must Long-term Services and Support demonstrate to apply for NCQA accreditation?
    a. Perform quality assessments
    b. Use generalized plans of care
    c. Address minor incidents only
    d. Manage transitions between LTSS and behavioral health services only

17. Which statement best defines the types of performance-based measures used by the NQF?
    a. Uses a unique set of performance-based measures that are not recognized by the state or federal level of government
    b. Utilizes a set of performance-based standards that are recognized by multiple groups including states, the federal government, and private sectors
    c. Does not utilize performance measures that can be leveraged to evaluate quality of care but instead is used in determining the quality of care coordination
    d. Favors performance-based measures that align to guidelines and standards that are only utilized in the private sector

18. What did the Joint Commission create to evaluate patient safety?
    a. National Patient Safety Goals
    b. Federal Patient Safety Goals and Guidelines
    c. National Patient Safety Goals and Standards
    d. National Patient Safety Goals and Measures

19. Which agency or group provides the opportunity for healthcare improvement by sharing research information that improves the accessibility, effectiveness, efficiency, and quality of healthcare that consumers receive?
    a. Agency for Healthcare Research and Quality (AHRQ)
    b. The Joint Commission
    c. National Committee for Quality Assurance (NCQA)
    d. URAC

20. What clearinghouse provides specific patient-centered outcomes that outline the MOST effective medical treatments for a particular condition based on current research?
    a. The National Standard Clearinghouse
    b. The National Guideline Clearinghouse
    c. The Independent Review Clearinghouse
    d. The U.S. Taskforce Guideline Clearinghouse

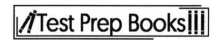

21. Which of the following is composed of sixteen national experts who independently provide evidence-based recommendations regarding the efficacy of preventive services that improve the health of Americans, including healthcare screenings, preventative medications, and primary care settings?
    a. NQA
    b. NCQA
    c. AHRQ
    d. USPSTF

22. How many stages of meaningful use are there associated with the HITECH Act?
    a. One
    b. Two
    c. Three
    d. Four

23. Which agency uses Quality Indicators (QIs) such as Patient Safety Indicators and Pediatric Safety Measures to measure the quality of healthcare, and may assist in the identification of quality concerns as well as identify areas of opportunity for additional research and study?
    a. AHRQ
    b. USPSTF
    c. NCQA
    d. NQF

24. Which of the following are examples of financial indicators?
    a. Cost effectiveness and cost savings
    b. Case manager tasks and activities
    c. Health risk assessments
    d. Mortality reporting

25. How is case management productivity measured?
    a. Time, tasks, and activities
    b. Length of stay, admissions, and readmissions
    c. Encounters, admissions, and readmissions
    d. Revenue, encounters, and admissions

26. Which of the following best describes the utilization quality indicator of daily census reporting?
    a. A summary of the average length of stay and number of and readmissions within 30 days
    b. An overview of budgeted inpatient days per 1000 to current inpatient days per 1000 with a seven- and 30-day trend
    c. Month-to-date and year-to-date encounters information by product line for both ambulatory and inpatient services
    d. A comparison of the benchmark length of stay detail to that of a given facility

27. Who can provide an organization with the client's experience?
    a. The physician
    b. The home health agency
    c. The client
    d. The hospital

Answer Explanations

1. C: The calculator is free of charge. The remaining answers are incorrect based on any reference to the calculator having a cost associated with it.

2. A: The four categories of the Caseload Matrix are as follows: initial elements impacting caseload, comprehensive needs assessment impacting caseload, case management interventions, and outcomes. The remaining answer choices are incorrect because they do not fall into the four categories as defined by the CMSA and NASW concept paper.

3. D: Cost-benefit analysis is the term that refers to how well an organization can show the value of a case management program. The remaining answer choices are incorrect. Health or medical benefit ratio (sometimes noted as the medical loss ratio) refers to the amount of premium revenue spent on medical care and services. Cost-effective comparison is not a term commonly used to show the value of a case management program.

4. B: The Mini-Mental State Examination is an example of a health risk assessment that is currently in use within various organizations. It is used to assess for cognitive function. The remaining options are incorrect. PDSA and Six Sigma are examples of quality improvement measurement strategies. The Case Mix Assessment Tool is not a standard assessment tool.

5. D: Predictive modeling is a tool that many organizations use to identify those people within their population who pose the greatest risk for preventable costs. The remaining answer options are incorrect. None of these terms are nationally recognized terms.

6. C: Most predictive models prefer to leverage 12 months of data to handicap the model. The remaining answer choices are incorrect. While 6 months is an option, it is not the preferred time frame, nor are the other answer choices.

7. A: Adjusted Clinical Groups. The remaining answer options are incorrect because they are not used to define the profile of a patient's morbidity as is seen with ACGs. They are not industry terms.

8. B: CQIs improve the overall quality of healthcare delivery therefore allowing for an identification of factors that affect healthcare outcomes. The remaining answer options are incorrect. They are not industry-recognized quality improvement programs.

9. A: Benchmarks can enable organizations to monitor trends and performance metrics in a consistent manner. The remaining answer options are incorrect because they are not a term that is commonly associated with monitoring the overall performance of a program.

10. A: URAC operates a case management accreditation program with a primary focus on enabling health plans to build a program that is actively capable of managing transitions. The remaining answer options are incorrect because they are not accrediting bodies.

11. B: URAC compares its measures with other reported measures from other entities such as AHRQ National Measures Clearing House and NQF. The remaining answers are incorrect. NCQA has HEDIS and NTOCC has a primary focus on the transition of patients between multiple healthcare settings and identifying gaps commonly seen that affect outcomes.

12. C: Organizations that fail to meet NCQA requirements during the Accreditation Survey are denied accreditation by NCQA. The remaining answers are incorrect based on this NCQA practice.

13. C: NCQA provides three categories of disease management accreditation: Accredited, Accredited with Performance Reporting, and Provisional Accreditation. Provisional accreditation alerts the industry that a disease management team does not meet all of the NCQA guidelines or standards, thus the remaining answers are incorrect.

14. A: NCQA utilizes HEDIS scores to measure the performance of managed care organizations. The remaining options are incorrect because HEDIS is the NCQA measure available to consumers to compare the performance of one health plan with another.

15. B: Organizations may be accredited for a three-year or a two-year duration by NCQA. The remaining options are incorrect based on this NCQA practice of a two- or three-year guideline.

16. A: Organizations that demonstrate the ability to achieve NCQA defined standards of managing transitions between levels of care or LTSS settings, performing quality individualized assessments, and the capacity to handle critical incidents may be eligible for NCQA accreditation. These are standards defined by NCQA and performed by LTSS organizations that would enable them to meet LTSS eligibility. The remaining options are incorrect. Care plans are not a component of eligibility defined by NCQA and as previously defined by the rationale, organizations must demonstrate a capacity to handle complex or critical situations commonly experienced within the LTSS population.

17. B: National Quality Forum uses a set of performance-based standards that multiple groups, including states, the federal government, and private sectors, recognize and utilize in the evaluation of the quality of performance and overall contribution to improving care. The remaining answer options are incorrect because they negate the overall role of the NQF as defined in the preceding statement.

18. A: National Patient Safety Goals (NPSGs) are created by the Joint Commission. These are standards that have the intention of improving patient safety across the healthcare continuum. The remaining answer options are not appropriate selections because the NPSGs are the only standards that are created by the Joint Commission.

19. A: The Agency for Healthcare Research and Quality (AHRQ) provides the opportunity for healthcare improvement in that it provides research information to the public and healthcare professionals. The remaining options are incorrect selections. NCQA and URAC are accrediting bodies. This is not the role of the Joint Commission.

20. B: The National Guideline Clearinghouse provides specific patient-centered outcomes and defines the medical treatments that are a best practice for a particular condition based on current research. The remaining options are incorrect. These guidelines do not exist.

21. D: The U.S. Preventive Task Force is a group of national experts who have responsibility to provide evidence-based recommendations that affect the health of Americans. This includes healthcare screenings, preventative medications, and primary care settings. The Task Force actually assigns letter grades to their recommendations, and cost is not considered when evaluating the effectiveness of the healthcare measure.

22. C: There are three stages of meaningful use and providers must demonstrate the ability to function within each of the stages before they can move to the next one. The remaining answers choices are incorrect based on the requirements of the HITECH Act for three stages.

23. A: AHRQ uses Quality Indicators to measure the quality of health care that supports the identification of quality concerns. The remaining answers options are incorrect because they are not the owners of the QI process. It is a function of AHRQ.

24. A: Cost effectiveness and cost savings are two commonly used financial indicators in quality measures by organizations to examine overall impact of services provided. The remaining answer options are incorrect. Neither of these are financial indicators used as a quality measure per se for an organization. Health risk assessments help to provide the patient's history, and mortality reporting is an outcome, not a financial indicator.

25. A: Data collection of productivity indicators for case managers may concentrate heavily on time, tasks, and activities. The remaining answer options are incorrect because they are more commonly associated with utilization indicators.

26. B: Utilization indicators are tracked to evaluate the effectiveness of case and disease management programs and to note the general trends and behaviors of the population that is being served. Industry-recognized utilization indicators that are measured include (but are not limited to) average length of stay, emergency department visits, readmissions within 30 days, and outpatient service utilization. Daily census reporting is a common utilization indicator. It provides an overview of budgeted inpatient days per 1000 to current inpatient days per 1000 with a seven- and 30-day trend. Choice A lists two other utilization indicators, but does not describe the specific utilization indicator of daily census reporting. Choice C describes encounters data, another utilization indicator, while Choice D describes the utilization indicator of average length of stay, not daily census reporting.

27. C: Client experience information can only come from the client or caregiver, although it may be collected by various entities such as the physician, hospital, or home health agency. The remaining options are incorrect because client experience information can only come from the client or caregiver.

Rehabilitation Concepts and Strategies

Certified case managers (CCMs) will invariably work with individuals requiring rehabilitative care in some form. Whether disabled due to a chronic or acute illness, all patients will benefit from CCM intervention and the formulation of an effective plan of care. One of the primary roles of the case manager is to act as an expert, maintaining a full awareness of the needs of the client, as well as the appropriate providers necessary to intervene. Acting as the collaborator, the clinician must form an interdisciplinary team of social workers, psychologists, physicians, physical and occupational therapists, and other ancillary staff to begin the plan for inpatient care and discharge. Through ongoing interaction, the CCM must continually collaborate with the client and interdisciplinary team members to develop a focused approach to manage the case.

When working in an inpatient unit, cases are primarily provided to the CCM through inpatient census reports. Without census reports, CCMs must hope to be alerted to new admissions by lurking in each unit or maintaining a perch in the emergency room. Alternatively, the clinician reviews the daily census periodically throughout the day as admissions occur, providing CCMs with up-to-the-minute information.

Checking with the charge nurse on each unit and checking the census report daily is helpful, but these techniques will not yield a full list of patients within the diagnosis-related groups (DRGs) that would likely benefit from CCM intervention. The primary DRGs typically referred to the CCM for rehabilitative intervention include but are not limited to: industrial accident victims, amputees, individuals with workplace injuries, burn victims, and those who have sustained a traumatic brain injury (TBI). Based on the census report, the CCM can decide which patients within these groups may need intervention and assistance with discharge planning. Typically, the CCM is responsible for ensuring the patient's appropriate level of care, proving consistent support, and guiding decision making to utilize and exhaust all available financial resources prior to discharge.

Most clients recovering from a workplace injury do plan to return to work, and most can do so within a short period of time. Little, if any, CCM involvement is required for clients with mild injuries or injuries outside of basic coordination of medical benefits to ensure coverage. However, clients who are unable to return to work as expected may face a longer road to recovery. The case manager will typically devote the majority of their time to preparing care plans and following up with clients affected by severe chronic illness and calamitous injuries.

For all of the aforementioned cases, the CCMs must be familiar with the myriad needs of these individuals. The necessary knowledge often includes available assistive devices, functional capacity assessments, ongoing needs post injury, acute versus chronic rehabilitation concepts, occupational rehab delivery systems, vocational considerations related to chronic illness, and permanent disability issues. Through supportive counseling, motivational interviewing, and a largely solution-focused approach, the client can slowly reach their goals. Overall, familiarity with the application of these concepts will be integral in the completion of a working care plan.

Adaptive Technologies

For individuals with pervasive or temporary injuries, it can be difficult for them to navigate their daily lives independently. The injury may also impact the client's ability to perform the duties of their occupation. In an effort to help clients return to a life that mirrors their previous level of functioning as closely as possible, assistive devices are often implemented. **Assistive devices** are utilized for short- or long-term use. Common types improve functional impairment (mobility and self-care aids) or augment sensory impairment (visual, auditory, speech devices). The primary objective is always to steer the patient toward the types of devices that engender self-confidence and increase self-reliance.

Depending on the type and severity of the patient's injury, several assistive devices may be required. The CCM must act as the collaborator and join forces with the patient and associated providers to determine: the type, severity, and impact of the injury; the type(s) of devices needed; and the estimated duration of the injury, which will be directly proportional to the overall costs incurred. For best practice, the CCM must also be knowledgeable of the safety, reliability, and pricing of the apparatus once it is deemed necessary. Acting again as an expert, the CCM must prepare to present the client with the available options. Collecting a list of similar items allows for comparable recommendations, freeing the patient to choose the most efficient and cost-effective devices whenever possible.

Once the list is compiled, the next step is to gauge the member's perceived versus actual needs related to assistive devices, as well as gain an understanding of the environment in which the desired items will be used. A basic understanding of the home and work environments, along with a basic blueprint of the floor plan is helpful. Appropriate questions include: Does the client live in a ranch-style, split-level, or multi level home? Is there an elevator in the workplace? How far is the client's bedroom from the main entry of the home? Are there any steps to navigate to enter the home and workplace? Does the workplace have wheelchair access or an elevator? How will toileting needs be addressed?

Numerous questions must be asked and answered in order to prepare the best plan for ongoing rehabilitative therapy and return to work. For example, individuals with acute disabilities don't necessarily have similar requirements. An individual who has a broken leg would likely need less recovery time and fewer assistive devices, and have a shorter expected recovery time, than an individual who has broken both legs. Although mobility is affected in both scenarios, the first individual would have an increased probability of performing basic self-care tasks than would someone with two broken legs. Handling crutches, although cumbersome, allows for the patient to navigate their home environment, while two broken legs would result in a bed-bound status, increasing the need for more assistive devices (toileting aids, transfer devices, dressing aids, wheelchair, etc.).

The most effective approach when working with these patients is to periodically assess their perceived needs and confirm that they are being met. As the patient recovers, their needs change and the prudent clinician must remain flexible and prepared to adjust the plan of care accordingly.

An individualized plan may reveal even more pertinent information. The same patient with one broken leg may be single, live alone, and have no social support, requiring additional help such as a folding cane chair. The clinician may need to locate a local service to provide assistance with house cleaning, grocery shopping, and other basic tasks that require more mobility than the member is capable of. Moreover, if that same individual lives in a multi-level home, with narrow halls or carpeting, and is also already physically frail, they may require a less imaginative care plan. Although having two broken legs denotes the need for extensive support, that individual may live with many caring and available family members, indicating less actual need for basic house cleaning and errands. If this same person lives in close quarters, has a shared bedroom, and is physically strong, their care plan would constitute fewer devices and more planning in other areas.

If possible, the case manager should consider the option of encouraging the client to attend support groups for individuals with similar prostheses. Perhaps that individual may also benefit from the clinician providing instruction to the caregiver regarding the needs of the patient. It is crucial, however, not to guide the client toward any specific decision. Self-determination is paramount in cases such as these, and the client must be allowed to decide if wearing a prosthetic device is an option to consider.

Injuries of a more serious and/or permanent nature will require equally permanent activity and daily living aids. Hearing aids, text telephone devices (TTD), teletypewriters (TTY), transfer devices (hydraulic lifts, modified or electric stair lifts), and augmentative and alternative communication devices (AAC) may be required. The injuries sustained may require the actual purchase of the items, rather than simply renting them.

An orthosis is an item used to correct, support, or improve declining muscle or limb function in a way that restores that function. Specifically, orthoses like braces must be purchased because they require customized design. A prosthesis actually replaces a missing limb or body part for both cosmetic and functional reasons. These two types of assistive devices must be produced by those specifically trained and certified to design, properly fit, and align them for each individual patient. The clinician will need to investigate the training of the prosthetist, the costs of the items, the available insurance coverage, and applicable state and federal assistance programs. A more comprehensive evaluation will likely be necessary in order to procure these items, as they typically require a prescription and assessment and/or evaluation by a licensed health care professional in the specific area of injury.

Functional Capacity Evaluation

Once the nature of the injury, required devices, and client needs are determined, an individualized assessment of the patient is also imperative. A typical **functional capacity assessment** includes an evaluation of an individual's ability to perform basic and job-specific tasks. An interdisciplinary team consisting of physicians, physical therapists (PTs), occupational therapists (OTs), and psychologists collaborate to interview, assess, and diagnose the patient in relation to their ability to perform the duties associated with their current job description and associated activities. The CCM's responsibility is to help locate the appropriate providers, facilitate the necessary appointments, and support the member through the assessment process. With the use of the necessary assistive devices, the member's functional threshold is established. Any deficits in functioning are addressed and, if required for a return to work, added to a PT or OT plan of care.

One of the objectives of the functional assessment is to answer several questions in relation to the injury: Can you do your job? Can you do your job in your current work environment? How well can you do your job in your current work environment? Are the assistive devices truly necessary? Are you able to manipulate the assistive devices, or are they too cumbersome?

The answers to the aforementioned questions help to build a simulation of the type of work environment, average daily tasks, and associated time frames. Baseline performance levels and endurance of treatment are obtained to be compared with the final assessment. Although maximum effort from the patient is expected, the assessment is not meant to be punitive or severe. The PT or OT will typically plan the activities to build upon themselves, progressing in difficulty as the client's mobility and/or range of motion improves. Barriers to the achievement of the most favorable outcome are identified, and strategies to intervene and correct the problems are developed. Once completed, the inventories will guide further intervention and assist the care team in recommending the individual for a return to work.

The clinician must also assess the client's needs as the client perceives them. Do the devices provide aid or support their ability to accomplish the tasks of daily living? Does the patient feel they can perform the necessary tasks with only the devices provided? Has the client considered an alternate occupation if a return to work is not obtained? How supportive is the client's home environment? What, if any, emotional or psychological deficits need to be met? How best can the CCM support the client in working through those concerns? Is the client willing or able to seek out other sources of emotional support through this process?

The answers to these questions are also crucial, as the treatment plan can be adjusted. If the client's needs have changed during the assessment process, those needs can be addressed and added to the plan of care. Whenever necessary, the clinician should involve the family and caregivers in the discussion, so that their concerns can also be addressed. Upon the completion of the final report, the case manager will then guide the member's return to work, with any assistive devices, prostheses, or orthotics deemed necessary for the member to perform at an optimal level of functioning.

Rehabilitation assessment tools are presented in the following table.

Functional Domains	Tools
Activities of Daily Living (ADL)	Barthel Index (Mahoney and Barthel 1965) FIM™ Instrument (Uniform Data System for Medical Rehabilitation 1997) Katz Index (Katz, et al., 1963) LIFEware℠ System (Baker, et al., 1997)
Ambulation/Locomotion	Dynamic Gait Index (DGI) (Jonsdottir and Cattaneo 2007) Functional Ambulation Profile (FAP) (Nelson 1974) Gait Abnormality Rating Scale (GARS) (Wolfson, et al., 1990) Physical Performance Battery (Guralnik, et al., 1994) Six Minute Walk (Butland, et al., 1982) Timed Up & Go (Podsiadlo and Richardson 1991) Walking Speed (Graham, et al., 2008)
Balance	Berg Balance Scale (Berg, et al., 1989) Balance Self-Perceptions Test (Shumway-Cook, et al., 1997) Functional Reach Test (Duncan, et al., 1990)
Cognitive Functioning	Mini-Mental-State Exam (MMSE) (Folstein, et al., 1975)
Depression	Beck Depression Inventory (BDI) (Beck, et al., 1988) Center for Epidemiologic Studies Depression Scale (CES-D) (Radloff 1977)
Executive Functioning	Stroop Test (Stroop 1935) Trails A & B Tests (Reitan 1955)
Instrumental Activities of Daily Living (IADL)	Everyday Problems Test (EPT) (Willis, et al., 1992) Lawton Index (Lawton and Brody 1969) LIFEware℠ System (Baker, et al., 1997) Pfeffer Index (Pfeffer, et al., 1982)
Memory	Wechsler Memory Scale (Tulsky and Ledbetter 2000)
Pain	McGill Pain Questionnaire (Melzack 1975) Visual Analog Scale (Revill, et al., 1976)
Well-Being/Health-Related Quality of Life (HRQOL)	36-Item Short-Form Health Survey (SF-36®) (Ware and Sherbourne 1992) Sickness Impact Profile (SIP) (Bergner, et al., 1981)

Rehabilitation Post Hospitalization or Acute Health Condition

Once the functional assessment has been completed with the necessary assistive devices, the next step is to formulate the care plan. At all times, the team must consider how the client will manage their lives in their home and work environments. The interdisciplinary team will determine which type of therapy is best suited to achieve optimal functioning. Equally important is the type of injury. Whether the injury requires occupational therapy or physical therapy, all injuries will require a rehabilitation regimen. Generally, workplace injuries are characterized as minor/mild, moderate, severe/calamitous, or fatal.

The majority of minor/mild occupational injuries include cuts and bruises, and may require only a brief urgent-care visit. Rehabilitative therapy, if necessary, can typically begin within days and is more likely to be short term. These patients are usually able to return to work quickly with little interruption of, or adjustments to, their workflow and environment. The utilization of assistive devices is often minimal and temporary. Also included in the mild category are repetitive injuries. The most familiar repetitive injury is carpal tunnel syndrome. Largely related to typists, hairdressers, and others who predominantly use their hands in repetitive motions, these patients can move swiftly into the moderate category if they continue to work in the same occupation. The CCM will work with all of these members to determine how quickly they can return to work and utilize their paid time off (PTO) to offset any time away from work (TAFW) as needed. These cases typically require less intervention.

When a workplace injury is moderate, requiring an ambulance transport and/or emergency room visit, more extensive planning and follow up are required. Moderate injuries can include, but are not limited to: slip and falls, sprains, strains, back injuries, and broken bones. Although these types of injuries will require immediate medical attention, once stabilized, these patients usually are able to return to work within a short, specified amount of time.

The case manager can advocate for the member to receive Family Medical Leave (FMLA) if necessary, and supplemental pay for TAFW. Other state and federal legislation such as the Consolidated Omnibus Budget Reconciliation Act (COBRA) may be applicable in cases like these. The application of the rules of COBRA would provide the client with continued medical benefits should they be unable to return to work.

For rehabilitative purposes, these patients will usually be given a list of restrictions and exercises to complete while recovering briefly at home. The essential work tasks to complete are the general focus of these interventions. The patient will meet with the physical therapist, occupational therapist, and/or physician to retrieve a "return to work" memorandum once cleared.

As the fatal injury requires no rehabilitative efforts, the next most significant area of concern for the CCM is the enormous classification of serious/catastrophic injury. For severe/calamitous occupational injuries, the member will not only need immediate medical attention, but a hospital admission for observation and additional treatment. The CCM's responsibility is to work in partnership with the patient, family members, and interdisciplinary team at the hospital in order to formulate the best short-term and long-term plan of care. A short list of these types of injuries includes: closed/open head injuries, machine-related crushing accidents, inclement-weather exposure, chemical-related accidents/spills, and electrocutions. Once the client's overall level of functioning is gauged, this will guide the CCM, patient, family members, and inpatient team to determine the most appropriate level of post-discharge care.

Unfortunately for patients requiring rehabilitative services after their initial medical hospitalization, the road to recovery is long and arduous. Workplace injuries and acute-illness management are treated similarly. An innumerable number of diagnostic tests and periodic functional assessments will occur during their inpatient stay in rehab. The CCM will work together with the inpatient team to periodically assess the patient's progress and adjust the care plan as needed. All aspects of daily living will be assessed regarding the patient's ability to perform self-care tasks and the degree to which that individual is prepared to return to the community. Emotional, physical, sensory, and processing deficits are also targeted.

These patients will receive a specialized discharge plan intended to complement their current level of independence. The majority of their rehabilitative discharge plan of care will act as scaffolding, remaining in place until the individual has been returned to an optimal level of functioning. For example, an individual who experienced a traumatic brain injury (TBI) as a result of a fall or industrial accident would likely be cared for initially in a regular hospital until cleared by their physician to undergo the intensive therapies of a rehabilitation center or hospital. Once the physical injuries have healed, the next task is to focus on the emotional, physical, and sensory aspects of the injury. Many of these patients experience substantial memory loss, poor coordination or spatial recognition, inability to process language or ideas, and difficulty verbalizing feelings or ideas.

For example, an individual with a frontal-lobe injury will likely experience difficulties with aggression or promiscuity. Damage in this area often results in a failure to inhibit emotions. If asked to make a sandwich, the individual may become overwhelmed with the details of the task, responding with frustration. Whereas someone without a TBI may become frustrated, they would likely possess the ability to inhibit a reflexive aggressive outburst. An individual with a cerebellar brain injury may be unable to hold the tools necessary to even complete the task.

Depending on the types of skills that need to be relearned, the CCM must continually support the patient and the family, providing assurance of the care plan while also delivering a realistic evaluation of the member's progress. Recovery for these patients can be slow, frustrating, and confusing. Periodic discussions regarding the client's motivation to continue are often required. These patients tend to require extensive services and ongoing rehabilitation either on an outpatient basis or with subsequent transfer to their home setting, an assisted-living facility, a subacute rehabilitative facility, or long-term skilled nursing care. Each treatment milieu builds from its predecessor, slowly integrating the member back into society.

Vocational and Rehabilitation Service Delivery Systems

For the vast majority of more serious cases, the patient will likely continue to receive extensive evaluation once discharged from the hospital. It is incumbent upon the CCM to ensure that this care continues uninterrupted; for this to occur, payment of the required services must be obtained. Individuals receiving rehabilitative services are engaged in a "system" consisting of a group of health care providers, the actual care setting, and the services themselves. This system implies that the community as a whole must be integrated into the care plan. All aspects of the patient's life must be reviewed in regard to the new disability. Care coordination with the correct entities is vital at this stage. Care can be delivered on a fee-for-service basis, through tele-health, managed care, or self-directed care.

In a **fee-for-service system**, providers are paid based on the specific services they provide. Each instance is paid separately, with reimbursement commensurate with the federally acceptable guidelines. This type of care is considered to be the most traditional and is utilized most often. It is performed in-person and occurs at some point throughout the life of every case. For example, providers are generally reimbursed for diagnostic tests, office visits, consultations, and specific procedures.

Tele-health is quickly becoming one of the most popular modalities with both health professionals and patients. The use of technology in the provision of health care is both convenient and cost effective. Patient-provider interactions are conducted over the telephone or through the computer. Members self-report symptoms, concerns, and reactions to medications or services.

Managed health care delivery involves an organization enlisted to monitor the costs and utilization of care. The managed-care organization (MCO) serves as the gatekeeper, with a predetermined allotment for services per member, otherwise known as capitation. Through applying capitation, MCOs preserve resources and prevent misuse or abuse of those resources.

These systems of delivery have two important functions. First, at the federal level, certain services are categorized as mandatory. These types of services represent basic care needs, are nonnegotiable, and include inpatient and outpatient hospitalization, in-home services, and family planning. Second, there is an allowance for the states to determine which non compulsory services will be covered. Some of the features of the latter include podiatric care, optometry, and chiropractic care. Unfortunately, physical and occupational therapies are also on the list of optional services. The CCM must work in collaboration with the member's medical insurer and health care providers to coordinate payment for services. Whenever possible, the clinician must act as an advocate on behalf of the client to maintain the continuity of care.

Vocational Aspects of Disability(ies) and Illness

The **Americans with Disabilities Act** (ADA) expressly forbids discrimination by employers toward the hiring, firing, or unequal treatment of any individual with a qualifying disability. This prohibition includes accessibility to: education, transportation, employment, public places, and recreational activities. Any employer found to be in violation of the ADA can face a minimum fine in civil cases of $55,000 and a maximum of $150,000.

Formally, a **disability** is defined as a psychological or medical condition that reduces a person's functional capacity in at least one area of the body. When a client with a disability is returning to work, they will likely need accommodations in order to perform their job. To ensure the client's return to work, the CCM must compare the functional assessment to the formal job description of the client. It is crucial to utilize the functional assessment at this stage and ensure the employer does not alter expectations and prevent the client's return to work. If, upon comparison of the essential job functions and the functional assessment, the CCM is able to determine that the client does qualify as disabled, the next step is to arrange reasonable accommodations.

At times, even after completing physical and occupational therapies, the client is not yet ready to return to work, even if accommodations are provided. For example, a bus driver recovering from injuries related to a vehicular accident may have regained the use of their extremities after traditional treatment, but residual injuries may still remain. That same individual may continue to suffer from chronic back pain from sitting and driving for hours, or experience anxiety or post-traumatic stress disorder (PTSD), including flashbacks of the incident when driving or in a vehicle.

To ease an individual back into the physical demands of their job, ergonomics may be used. Ergonomics is the science of matching the physical requirements of a job to the physical abilities of the worker. Musculoskeletal injuries can occur if physical demands are greater than the employee's physical capabilities. Body mechanics refers to how the body moves during activities of daily living. Understanding and practicing the use of proper body mechanics is imperative to preventing injury. Ergonomic devices such as special seat pads, back braces, or pillows can be provided to ease physical demands and reduce the risk of injury. If these additions do not cause relief, more therapies may be required. In this instance, a work-hardening program is the next logical step.

Also referred to as "functional restoration" or "work conditioning," work-hardening programs were created as a bridge between where the medical treatment ends and where the client's work environment begins. The CCM must assemble a team from a variety of specialties: ergonomics, prosthetics, physical and occupational therapy, and psychology. With the team in place, it is also necessary to confirm that the employer agrees to allow the client to return to work. The CCM must confirm the client knows they will not be forced to return to work unprepared. Although the client may be emotionally ready to return to work, they may not be physically able to do so. The goal is to provide a simulated work environment and gradually reintroduce the client to specific tasks and activities directly associated with the position they will be returning to.

In the above example, the member may be asked to sit, with the use of the ergonomic assistive devices (such as a specially designed chair or chair pad), for minutes, then hours, gradually building up to the specified time expected to complete a shift. The psychologist on the team can then work directly with the member to address PTSD and/or anxiety through cognitive behavioral therapy, positive self-talk, or affirmations. Throughout the duration of the treatment, the team will be working toward the goal of helping the member reach the functional capability to return to work.

Rehabilitation Concepts

As case managers attempt to move their patients along the continuum of care, they should be familiar with rehabilitation concepts. A major role of case managers is to educate patients on their available benefits so that they will be able to receive services whenever they move to the next step along the continuum.

The case manager should have a working knowledge of what qualifies a patient for inpatient versus outpatient rehabilitation. For patients to qualify under CMS for inpatient medical rehabilitation facilities, patients must be able to actively participate in multiple therapies for a total of three hours per day, five days per week, with providers documenting the benefits they expect to see from this rehabilitation.

The case manager must evaluate the patient and know the most appropriate types of facilities available for referral. For example, many medical rehabilitation facilities require that patients are not ventilator dependent and that they do not require urinary catheterization frequently as part of their guidelines for admission. The case manager must work with the patient, family, the provider, and the rest of the disciplinary team to present rehabilitation options that the family can choose from.

Vocational rehabilitation is an individualized program for employment which is designed to help patients with a disability return to the labor force. Vocational rehab includes services such as counseling, training, job placement, assistive technology, and career exploration. Each state offers different services and some include independent living programs, so case managers should be aware of services offered in their state to help make appropriate referrals.

Substance use rehabilitation may be needed for patients at many points along the continuum. Funding for substance use rehab is often a difficult hurdle to overcome and varies greatly state by state. If patients have health insurance, contacting the insurer for possible participating facilities may be useful. Case managers should be aware of local substance use rehabs. Some rehabs accept Medicare and Medicaid, and some facilities are willing to charge on a sliding scale for fees. The U.S. Department of Health and Human Services offers the SAMHSA website, which has a behavioral health treatment services locator. Case management services are needed for patients with substance use disorder because these patients often suffer further from lack of coordinated services and other health and social problems.

Practice Questions

1. How are cases provided to the CCM on an inpatient unit?
    a. By periodically checking with the charge nurse on each unit.
    b. Through a daily check of the hospital census report.
    c. Requesting that the charge nurse of each unit page or call the CCM upon each admission.
    d. By periodically checking the daily census report for all admissions throughout the day.

2. Which of the following is included in the assessment of the need for assistive devices?
    a. The type of injury sustained by the client.
    b. The cost of the specific assistive device
    c. Whether the client was injured at work or at home
    d. If the client believes that they can recover from the injury.

3. Eric has sustained an injury that may require the use of a prosthetic limb. Which of the following would NOT be included in preparation for counseling the patient?
    a. Consult with a prosthetist specifically trained and certified to design and fit the required prosthetic.
    b. Locate a support group for patients with similar prostheses and/or amputations.
    c. Advise the client that the prosthetic device is the best choice for mobility.
    d. Compile a list of available options to present to the client for consideration.

4. What is the purpose of an orthosis?
    a. To replace a missing limb or body part for both cosmetic and functional reasons.
    b. To heal a limb or body part post injury.
    c. To support or improve declining muscle or limb function.
    d. To prevent an injury to a limb or body part.

5. A case manager has been asked to work on a team to evaluate a client post rehabilitation. The client has been fitted with a prosthetic but has been unable to return to work due to what he reports as "just not feeling right." What group of functional domain assessments should be considered for individuals who are experiencing chronic pain of an unknown origin after injury?
    a. Berg Balance Scale; Balance Self-Perceptions Test; Functional Reach Test.
    b. Timed Up and Go; Physical Performance Battery; Gait Abnormality Rating Scale.
    c. Beck Depression Scale; Depression Scale; Mini Mental Exam.
    d. None of the above.

6. What types of behaviors can be expected from an individual with a frontal-lobe injury?
    a. Poor balance and impaired depth perception.
    b. Promiscuity and low frustration tolerance.
    c. Difficulty recognizing words and progressive blindness.
    d. Poor fine motor skills and gait impairment.

7. Which of the following would be considered a moderate workplace injury?
    a. Repetitive injuries
    b. Cuts and bruises
    c. Broken bones
    d. Electrocutions

8. Which of the following is true of a functional capacity evaluation?
    a. It includes an evaluation of the ability to perform basic and job-specific tasks.
    b. A team approach is not utilized.
    c. The treatment plan is created and must remain the same throughout rehabilitation.
    d. Minimum effort from the client is all that is expected.

9. Jane's husband, Tom, has suffered a traumatic brain injury (TBI). How should the CCM counsel her regarding the concerns of recovery?
    a. The caregivers must expect the client to recover quickly.
    b. The client should be placed in an institution for his own safety.
    c. Every client with a TBI will have similar symptoms.
    d. The caregiver must expect specific deficits and plan how to handle them.

10. What is ergonomics?
    a. The study of how assistive devices affect an individual's quality of life.
    b. The science of creating effective ways to prepare an individual to return to their home environment.
    c. The study of creating more efficient ways for people to work in their vocational environment.
    d. The science of teaching a client how to adjust to the outside world.

11. How should a CCM counsel a client with a total knee replacement (TKR) that does not wish to return to work despite the physical ability to do so?
    a. The CCM must advise the client that they must return to work because they agreed to do so in their treatment plan.
    b. The CCM must negotiate an alternate return to work date with the employer while attempting to help the client change their mind.
    c. Advise the client that their claim may not be covered if they do not return to work as agreed upon in their treatment plan.
    d. The CCM must discuss the client's hesitation for returning to work to determine if a slower part-time to full-time return to work is more reasonable.

12. Which of these is the MOST important factor of work-hardening programs?
    a. Making sure that the client is physically and emotionally prepared to return to work as soon as possible.
    b. To provide a simulated work environment to gradually reintroduce the client to specific tasks directly associated with the position that they will be returning to.
    c. Confirming that the client is still able to perform the specific work-related tasks of their job without assistance.
    d. Making sure that the client is aware that they may have to return to work before they feel ready to do so.

13. What is the primary goal of the CCM when working with clients requiring rehabilitation services?
    a. To work with a client to help them to return to their previous level of functioning.
    b. To work with the client until they no longer need ongoing case management.
    c. Making sure that the client feels ready to leave treatment.
    d. To work with the client until they are able to return to work.

14. Which diagnosis-related groups (DRGs) are NOT typically flagged for CCM intervention?
    a. Individuals who have sustained a TBI.
    b. Industrial accident victims.
    c. Amputees or possible amputees.
    d. Women with high-risk pregnancies.

15. Which of the following is NOT a basic rehabilitation delivery system?
    a. The self-directed-care delivery system.
    b. The group-care delivery system.
    c. The managed-care delivery system.
    d. The fee-for-service delivery system.

16. Which functional domain of assessment tools is BEST suited to evaluate a client with a cerebellar TBI?
    a. The group primarily targeting activities of daily living.
    b. The group of assessment tools that target executive functioning.
    c. The set of assessment tools primarily targeting the ambulation and locomotion.
    d. The group primarily targeting cognitive functioning.

Answer Explanations

1. D: This answer is correct because this strategy allows the CCM to periodically review the census report for new admissions, physician orders, and diagnoses related to prolonged admission. This way, the CCM can plan which units to round on and create a plan for how to follow up with each specific patient. Choice *A* is incorrect because the charge nurse is typically made aware of an admission within thirty minutes to one hour beforehand. This strategy also interrupts the continuity of care for other patients on the unit. The charge nurse has many other duties and likely patients to care for as well. Choice *B* is incorrect even though running the census report is the best way to determine which patients in a given DRG have been admitted. It is necessary to run this report periodically throughout the day to check for new admissions. Choice *C* is also incorrect. See rationale for *A*.

2. A: This answer is correct because the type of injury sustained by the client can initially help guide the intervention. The associated DRG typically has a critical pathway that the CCM can utilize for planning care before and after discharge. Choice *B* is incorrect. The overall cost of the device is not useful in assessing the need for such a device. Choice *C* is incorrect because the location of where the injury took place is not relevant to the need for the assistive device. Choice *D* is incorrect because while the client's beliefs about recovery are valid, those beliefs cannot guide the number and types of devices.

3. C: This answer is correct because the CCM must not impose what they believe to be the best option onto the client. Once informed consent is obtained, the CCM must allow the client to determine which option they feel most comfortable choosing. It is the client who must live with the results. Choice *A* is incorrect because the CCM must utilize the most highly trained and best equipped technician to design, align, and fit the prosthetic. This professional will use the client's medical, personal, and professional profile to design a device best suited for the client to use. Choice *B* is incorrect because the client may benefit from speaking with others with similar diagnoses, other amputees, or those with specific personal and/or work environments who can empathize with the client and help to normalize their questions and concerns. Choice *D* is incorrect because the client is entitled to choose the course of treatment that they prefer. Creating a list of appropriate devices and treatment plans will afford the client the information necessary to choose well.

4. C: This answer is correct. The goal of an orthosis is to improve the functioning of any body part and include but are not limited to shoe inserts, slings, and braces. Choice *A* is incorrect; this is a definition of a prosthetic. Choice *B* is incorrect because the orthosis does not heal any body part. Choice *D* is incorrect because the orthosis is not designed to prevent injuries.

5. C: This answer is correct because the client appears to be suffering from depression. The associated inventories are designed to gauge the client's mood and determine the level of depression. Choice *A* is incorrect. Although the client has sustained an injury that would likely affect their balance, the issue in this case is more related to a nonphysical cause. Choice *B* is incorrect. The client in this scenario does not report an ill fit, decline in mobility, or any changes in physical functioning. Choice *D* is incorrect.

6. B: This answer is correct because a frontal-lobe injury is an assault to the brain's primary emotion control center. The client will experience difficulties modulating emotions and struggle with inhibition. Choice *A* is incorrect. The behaviors noted in this selection are indicative of an injury to the temporal lobe. Choice *C* is incorrect and indicates an injury to the occipital lobe. Choice *D* is incorrect because it is indicative of an injury to the cerebellum.

7. C: Broken bones are considered a moderate workplace injury because while they necessitate a hospital visit, once treated, only require a short amount of time for recovery. Choices *A* and *B* are incorrect because these types of injuries would be categorized as minor or mild. Choice *D* is incorrect because electrocutions are included in the category of severe/calamitous occupational injuries.

8. A: This answer is correct because completing an evaluation of the ability of a client to perform basic and job-specific skills is the first step of a functional capacity evaluation. Choice *B* is incorrect. An interdisciplinary team is brought together to collaborate on the evaluation. Choice *C* is incorrect because treatment plans can be adjusted as necessary during the rehabilitation process. Choice *D* is incorrect because maximum effort is expected from the patient.

9. D: Working in tandem with the neurologist, the CCM must help the caregiver to understand the brain functions and the consequences of damage to any specific area. Choice *A* is incorrect because any client who has sustained a TBI will experience a myriad of symptoms and will likely never fully recover to their previous level of functioning. Choice *B* is incorrect. The client and caregiver must make this decision. The choice to permanently hospitalize a client is a delicate matter and, although it should be added to the plan as a viable option, the CCM must consider the needs of the patient and family as a unit. Choice *C* is incorrect. Depending on the specific area of damage, the client will experience many symptoms. Each area of the brain is responsible for a specific function; damage to any specific area will have a specific set of physical and/or emotional reactions.

10. C: Ergonomics is the study of creating more efficient ways for people to work in their vocational environment. Choice *A* is incorrect. Devices can be used within ergonomics to positively impact the client's life, but ergonomics is not defined as the study of assistive devices. Choice *B* is incorrect. Clients' return to their work environments is the paramount goal of ergonomics, rather than returning to their home environments. Choice *D* is incorrect. Ergonomics is not the science of teaching a client how to adjust to the outside world, but rather to their work environment.

11. D: The CCM must discuss the client's hesitation for returning to work to determine if a slower part-time to full-time return to work is more reasonable. Choice *A* is incorrect. The client can make adjustments to their treatment plan as needed. Choice *B* is incorrect. The CCM must allow the client to determine the best pace for treatment. Choice *C* is incorrect. The client's treatment plan must take into account the slow progression or even a setback in treatment.

12. B: This answer is correct. The CCM must reassure the client that the employer has agreed to allow the employee to be reintegrated into their previous work environment. Choice *A* is incorrect. The client will be assured that there will be sufficient time for them to relearn all of the hard and soft skills necessary to perform their job functions. Choice *C* is incorrect. Assistive devices will be utilized if necessary. Choice *D* is incorrect. The client will NOT be forced to return to work unprepared.

13. D: This answer is correct. The goal of the treatment plan is to guide the client's return to work. Choice *A* is incorrect. The client may never return to the level of functioning prior to their injury. Choice *B* is incorrect. The CCM is not to continue an intervention indefinitely, but to refer the client for ongoing services once their need for specific intervention has been satisfied. Choice *C* is incorrect. The client may never feel ready to leave treatment; the CCM must periodically advise the client on their progress and plan for the contract to end.

14. D: This answer is correct. Although these clients will benefit from CCM intervention, they are typically referred to an obstetrical specialist. Choice *A*, *B*, and *C* are incorrect. These types of clients are typically referred to a CCM due to the high probability of needing post hospitalization case management.

15. B: This answer is correct. There is no rehabilitation delivery system of this nature other than support groups, which are not a primary source of treatment. Choice *A* is incorrect. This delivery system allows for the client to care for themselves as often as possible, directing the course of treatment. Choice *C* is incorrect. This response refers to the insurance company acting as the primary gatekeeper of benefits. Choice *D* is incorrect. This type of care occurs after a face-to face interaction with a provider.

16. C: This answer is correct. A cerebellar injury typically results in an interruption of coordination, fine motor skills, ambulation, and the ability to grasp objects. Choice *A* is incorrect. These tools are designed to gauge balance. Choice *B* is incorrect. These tools are designed to gauge damage to the frontal lobe, where initiation, motivation and inhibition are housed. Choice *D* is incorrect. These tools are designed to gauge damage to the frontal lobe.

Ethical, Legal, and Practice Standards

For the certified case manager, it is vital to possess a working knowledge of the basics of employer, local, state, and federal requirements for the care and maintenance of individuals affected by workplace injuries. This knowledge, combined with evidence-based decision making, is integral in formulating an appropriate care plan and ensuring coverage for that care. Certain state and federal legislations require very specific accommodations for persons with disabilities, and benefits can be immediate. Specifically, all CCMs must at least be acquainted with the concepts of evidence-based practices regarding treatment guidelines, ethical considerations, regulatory requirements, privacy and confidentiality issues, risk management, and the overall scope of their practice.

Case Recording and Documentation

It is imperative that the CCM maintain immaculate and accurate case records. **Records** contain the chronological life of the case and provide a detailed description of and justification for services recommended and rendered. This is necessary due to a possible audit of the records by the responsible employer or other interdisciplinary team members and possible litigation. For example, if an employer decided to dispute the stipulations in a previously agreed upon return to work, the clinician can refer to the case file to negotiate. Accurate record keeping can also guide the interventions of an alternate CCM if the primary clinician is unavailable. Any planned or unexpected absence would not derail the progression of the case. Throughout the life of every case, the CCM will communicate with various providers, family members, and clients. Whenever possible, the CCM can record the sessions, as well as take notes, in an effort to ensure that no information is lost.

All case files require specific information to be considered complete. First, **basic demographic information** such as the client's name, past medical history, current diagnoses, medications, and contact information are required. Next, the clinician must **document the plan of care**, including the discharge plan and contingency plan if the patient decompensates unexpectedly. Also important to include in the client's case file is a **basic needs analysis**. The needs analysis is an outcropping of the functional assessment but also includes the client's perceived needs and hopes regarding the outcome of their treatment. As previously mentioned, all patient and provider communication is essential, with coinciding dates and times if available. Finally, it is crucial that the **cost of treatment** with and without case management be included. This is an extension of informed consent. This stipulation allows the client to consider the financial and medical advantages and disadvantages of working with the CCM and allows the client to make their decision based on all available information.

The certified case manager can maintain case-file information in various ways, like paper documents, audio or visual recordings, or a specific document management system (DMS). This type of record keeping utilizes a computer program that operates as a filing system. Several different formats exist with the goal of streamlining documentation while gleaning significantly more information to track clients' progress and outcomes and to later evaluate interventions. Reports can be quickly generated, and specific functions allow for multiple clients to be tracked for program evaluation purposes or trends with regards to diagnosis-related groups. These reports can then impact future interventions based on the successes garnered through work with similar clients.

In addition to the information in each specific client's file, the CCM must clearly delineate the supervision and/or consultation received on each case. This type of documentation shows that the clinician was not making decisions in a vacuum but in collaboration with other experienced colleagues. It is also important to cite all evidence-based bodies of knowledge, periodicals, seminars, articles, and books utilized in the care of clients. Providing verification that the interventions provided by the clinician are evidence based and current is both necessary and professional. Appropriate documentation of consultations helps to provide a clear and logical template of the plan of care if case files are audited.

Case managers frequently receive reports for the clients on their caseload. The majority of these reports include: a copy of the proposed plan of care, the client's progress with treatment, any actual barriers to achieving the necessary tasks to complete the plan of care, solutions to remove any deficits in functioning, and current cost analysis. These reports allow for the CCM to observe the client's progress over time, recognize any trends, and communicate effectively regarding the care plan with the patient and interdisciplinary team.

Ethics Related to Care Delivery

When providing consultation and case management, the CCM will inevitably encounter cases that present an ethical dilemma. Some of the most common dilemmas presented to the CCM include the client's refusal of services/treatment, experimental treatments and protocols, and end-of-life decisions. In these types of situations, the CCM must weigh the advantages and disadvantages of the proposed treatment in order to guide the patient to make an informed decision.

One of the preferred techniques to utilize when working with clients is motivational interviewing. This method is especially effective when working with clients who are struggling with ambivalence, or indifference, to beginning treatment. **Motivational interviewing** is a coaching technique that involves asking a series of open-ended and probing questions while summarizing the client's responses. As the client responds to the questions, their motivations and most desirable outcomes are clarified. The client's own words become the primary tool for building the plan of care. The CCM must also affirm the client's ability to verbalize their own goals. The main objective of this technique is to use the client's own words to help determine if the plan actually aligns with their verbalized goals.

Encountering the **refusal of treatment** by a client can be difficult to navigate. It is the task of the CCM to evoke not only the client's reason for declining treatment but to also determine what other options, if any, exist that would guide the client to a similar or more desirable outcome. For example, consider the dilemma of working with a patient that experienced a crushing injury that required a total left-knee replacement (TKR) who is also a Jehovah's Witness. For the majority of patients who undergo TKR, post-operative blood transfusions are warranted. It is widely known that Jehovah's Witnesses do not accept allogenic, or blood from a compatible donor, transfusions. Typically, the CCM would have the benefit of basic demographic information, including gender, marital status, and religious affiliations.

In this circumstance, the CCM would need to prepare an alternative intervention for the client, prior to the presentation. Enlisting the assistance of the orthopedic surgeon and hematologist, the CCM would be able to determine if autologous, or collection and reinfusion of the client's own blood components, would be an acceptable option. Once an alternative to the traditional option of allogenic blood transfusion is prepared, both can be presented to the client. In so doing, the clinical care team is not only providing full disclosure, they are also practicing with an open awareness of their client's religious convictions. Ultimately, it is the client who must decide the result; the CCM must honor that choice as long as there is no harm to come to the client as a result of that choice.

An additional ethical dilemma encountered by the CCM directly related to rehabilitative medicine is the decision of whether or not to utilize experimental treatments. Consider the same patient with a crushing knee injury. For this example, the individual is not a Jehovah's Witness and did agree to receive the transfusion. This client must weigh the decision of accepting a traditional prosthetic limb versus living life with a transplanted cadaver limb. The CCM in this situation must consider the client's autonomy, allowing the patient to determine which option to accept. Consideration of the client's hesitance to accept a cadaver limb is crucial. The CCM may suggest that the client attend support groups for amputees, consider only being counseled on the available research involving the transplantation of the cadaver limb, or talking with their clergy for spiritual guidance.

For end-of-life versus palliative-care concerns, especially where no advance directives are present, the CCM must follow state statutes and consult the legal next of kin. When advance directives are present, the CCM must preserve the client's autonomy and honor their wishes.

Ethics Related to Professional Practice

Certified case managers are required by the dictates of their licensing board to provide compassionate, ethical, and professional care at all times. The **Case Management Society of America** (CMSA) formulated a specific plan to address ethical concerns routinely faced by CCMs.

The **five basic ethical principles** are shown in the following graphic.

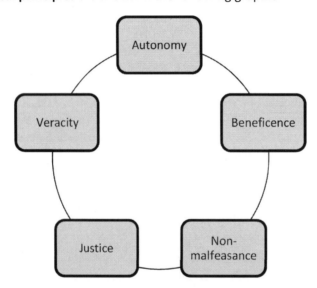

The generous application of these guiding principles is crucial to maintain a cohesive relationship between the CCM and the client. Although every human being has their own personal biases, morals, and values, the clinician must cast them aside, as much as possible, in order to provide clinically competent care. For the CCM, the roles of professional, advocate, communicator, and clinically competent collaborator come into focus.

Certified case managers must always conduct themselves in a professional manner. More importantly, it is vital that the CCM practices within the law. In order to do this, the clinician must obtain prior informed consent from the client or other responsible party. To be valid, the informed consent must contain a full explanation of the information needed to provide support, allow for the patient to specify a time frame for which the agreement is in effect, and evidence the signature of a third party to confirm the patient was not in duress at the time the contract was signed. It is the responsibility of the CCM to periodically evaluate the client's comfort level with the services received and confirm that expectations for ongoing care are clearly outlined.

Once the initial plan of care is agreed upon, the first step is for the CCM to enlist the member to identify their most crucial needs. By encouraging the member to be **autonomous**, the clinician is placing the client in the position to develop the confidence necessary to trust themselves to articulate their needs effectively. The member may articulate emotional issues or concerns that require the intervention of a psychologist for ongoing psychotherapy and/or prescribed medications. This strategy also teaches the member how to develop an internal locus of control, leading to the establishment of a foundation of self-confidence on which to build. During this process, the stage of change that the member is grappling with becomes clear. Having moved beyond precontemplation, through contemplation and goal-setting in the preparation phase, the member is slowly steered into action. In this instance, the clinician is acting in the roles of both communicator and advocate, placing the client in the position to utilize their own voice in setting the goals for recovery.

Both **beneficence** and **non-malfeasance** are closely related. It is not enough to provide empathetic and compassionate care. The CCM must also continually evaluate the plan of care so as not to inadvertently cause harm. The notion of **justice** combines the ideas behind beneficence and non-malfeasance, along with practicing in an ethically sound manner. Fundamental to every relationship is the expectation of fair treatment. There are additional considerations for the CCM regarding ethical service delivery. The expectation of receiving appropriate care is bolstered by the trust that has developed from previous interactions with the clinician. Acting as a collaborator, the CCM is focused on guiding the client to work toward viable solutions and to act. Practicing **veracity** is simply providing solution-focused options that are grounded in reality and truth. This technique is more pronounced in the relationship between the client and the CCM as time passes. Further, because of the trust required by the client to allow another individual to guide their decisions, failure to be authentic can result in a breakdown in the patient-client relationship.

Health Care and Disability Related Legislation

An innumerable amount of state and federal mandates, policies, and regulations govern how patients are to receive rehabilitative services. Other legislation was adopted to monitor the administration of financial support. The CCM must actively navigate the applicable statutes for each client and manage the team's approach to exhausting all available benefits. The myriad number of disability and health care laws will not be discussed in full, but additional information can be found at https://www.disability.gov/health-related-laws/. Some of the most notable statutes regarding disability are discussed below.

Americans With Disabilities Act (ADA)

The **Americans with Disabilities Act** (ADA) is one of the most significant pieces of legislation relating to persons with disabilities is Section 504 of the Rehabilitation Act of 1973. This civil rights legislation prohibits discrimination against persons with disabilities in programs that receive federal funding and led to the creation of the Americans With Disabilities Act (ADA) of 1990. The ADA was enacted to enforce strict sanctions on those who discriminate against persons who have a documented history of a disability, are viewed as having a disability, or are diagnosed with a mental or physical condition that has resulted in functional impairment. The prudent clinician will utilize the ADA when securing appropriate accommodations for their patients.

Family Medical Leave Act of 1993 (FMLA)

The Family Medical Leave Act of 1993 (FMLA) was written to allow for individuals to take an unpaid leave of absence to care for ill family members for a maximum of twelve weeks per calendar year while pre-servicing their medical benefits at up to 102% of the cost of their original employer premium.

The Health Insurance Portability and Accountability Act of 1996 (HIPAA)

The **Health Insurance Portability and Accountability Act** of 1996 (HIPAA) was enacted to remedy a number of issues faced by American citizens seeking medical coverage. This law provides the following: **Title I** focuses on portable health benefits, meaning that individuals with pre-existing conditions cannot be fired or lose coverage when renewing benefits; **Title II** is meant to curtail fraud and abuse of power by insurance companies and imposes strict requirements that personal health information be protected and confidential; **Title III** created optional savings accounts designed to offset medical care costs and lowered the cost of annual premiums paid by consumers; **Title IV** authorizes the Office of Civil Rights to enforce all provisions of this law; and **Title V**, "Revenue offsets" deals with regulations on how employers can deduct company-owned life insurance premiums for income tax purposes.

Workforce Innovation and Opportunity Act of 2014 (WIOA)

The establishment of the **Workforce Innovation and Opportunity Act** WIOA improved upon the Workforce Investment Act of 1998 and resulted in provisions to increase vocational training and job placement for disabled individuals. The clinician's application of the rules within this legislation is crucial in securing a return to work for clients.

Employee Retirement Income Security Act of 1974 (ERISA)

The **Employee Retirement Income Security Act** (ERISA) is a federal law that seeks to ensure that insurance companies adhere to very strict turn-around times when processing disability claims. Although the initial intent was to standardize basic coverage for disabled persons, this act has expanded over time to serve as a platform for insurers to deny coverage, as long as that denial of benefits falls within the law. Clients usually have to file an appeal in writing to any denied claim for medical benefits within sixty days of receiving the notification in the mail. Any claims submitted after that time do not legally have to be honored. The CCM must be aware of this common tactic to initially deny disability claims and pursue an appeal and exhaust the appeals process.

COBRA

Clinicians must also be familiar with the **Consolidated Omnibus Budget Reconciliation Act** (COBRA) of 1986. This piece of legislation allows individuals to maintain their medical benefits in the event of unexpected loss of employment, whether voluntary or involuntary. The employer bears the responsibility of notifying the client of their eligibility for COBRA once employment is terminated. Notification generally occurs within two weeks after job loss. The enrollment period is sixty days and is a continuation of the employer's elected benefits packages, including dental, vision, medical. The advantage to the client is that they can elect to maintain only the specific coverage that they need.

Specifically related to rehabilitation, this act allows for the employee, spouse, or dependent children to continue to receive medical coverage for a minimum of eighteen months and a maximum of thirty-six months. However, the premiums must be paid and can reach as much as 102% of the annual premium. Premature termination of this benefit can occur if the premiums are unpaid, the client becomes eligible for Medicare, the employer is unable to maintain the group plan, or the client acquires alternate employer-based coverage.

Mental Health Parity Act Rehabilitation Act of 1996

Mental Health Parity Act Rehabilitation Act of 1996 was established to prevent the discrimination against individuals with mental health problems. This is a federal law that strictly prohibits placing financial caps of mental health treatments unless those same limits also apply to medical benefit coverage.

Occupational Safety and Health Administration (OSHA)

OSHA began in 1970 as a way to enforce occupational safety concerns. OSHA works together with certain parts of the Americans with Disabilities Act to ensure that employees have rights, protection and compensation.

Affordable Care Act

The **Patient Protection and Affordable Care Act** (PPACA), often referred to as **Obamacare**, ensures that all patients receive the necessary health care services at reasonable costs. Conceptualized by President Barack Obama, the PPACA was officially declared law on March 23, 2010. The law created an open marketplace in which patients are free to choose from a variety of different insurers, intended to exemplify capitalism at its best. The PPACA was not only developed to provide American citizens with appropriate health care, no matter their financial status, it was also created to aid small-business owners by providing an incentivized system. Individuals are able to secure basic medical benefits through their employer, directly through insurance companies, or in the health insurance marketplace. These marketplaces, or health care exchanges, create an opportunity for clients and their families to obtain the most affordable coverage with fewer opt-out clauses for insurers.

A specific website, or portal, was developed to allow easy access to compare the different plans. Once the individual enters their demographic and financial information into the system, they are presented with several appropriate and comparable coverage options. The PPACA was enacted to ensure certain benefits are treated as indispensable. They include but are not limited to: maternity and infant care; dental and vision care; hospitalizations; emergent and outpatient services; mental health; preventative care; and rehabilitative services. When the client chooses their preferred plan, they are allowed to access the associated hospitals, providers, and physicians that have agreed to provide care to the patients that have chosen that particular health care plan, also known as the "network."

Since its beginning, the PPACA has been challenged in court for its constitutionality. In 2012, the provision that stated citizens must have a minimum level of health insurance or pay a penalty was upheld in NFIB v. Sebelius. The 2017 Tax Cuts and Jobs Act changed the payment that the provision required for failure to maintain insurance to zero dollars. This led to a group of states, led by Texas, to again challenge the PPACA, in a case known as California vs. Texas. In December of 2019, The U.S Court of Appeals for the 5th circuit ruled that that provision was unconstitutional. The Supreme Court will now review the decision to decide whether reducing the amount of minimum coverage to zero makes this unconstitutional, and if so, can that provision be removed from the rest of the PPACA. If the PPACA is removed, the consequences could include elimination of subsidies that makes insurance cost less, decreased eligibility for Medicaid, and removal of protections for patients that have preexisting conditions.

HITECH Act

The Health Information Technology for Economic and Clinical Health Act (HITECH), introduced in 2009, had the goal of promoting electronic health records. The act gave incentives to encourage providers to make the change to electronic health records, as well as increasing penalties for those found violating HIPAA.

As previously mentioned, the CCM often utilizes electronic health records (EHR) to document care provided to patients. Other health care professionals also contribute to the client's medical record. Although the maintenance of a client's records must be secure and private, there are other considerations. Record keeping is not meant to simply show what was accomplished in any given case. The record keeping must also present the purpose of the initiation of the case and how the introduction of the CCM added value to that case.

The clinician is expected to show that their participation in the client's treatment closed the apparent gaps in care and that the CCM identified previously unknown or unattended gaps in care. The purpose of the Meaningful Use Clause (a part of HITECH) created not only a clearinghouse of information that all providers can access, but also required providers to verify that the use of the database results in improved outcomes for patients. HITECH also held businesses associated with healthcare that had access to medical records accountable to HIPAA standards. They became legally required to protect PHI and could now face civil or criminal penalty for failure to do so.

Widespread use of the EHR has resulted in a more efficient and cost-effective health care model. Practitioners can now present their value to the case. By showing that their interventions have both quantitative and qualitative value, they justify continuing to provide that care. Along with the inception of the EHR came changes in coding for patient treatment and penalties for the failure to adhere to basic standards of practice. Since the HITECH act, now at least 96% of acute care hospitals have implemented EHRs.

Legal and Regulatory Requirements Applicable to Case Management Practice

In this litigious society, the prudent case manager must be diligent in their provision of care. It is not enough to simply follow basic practice standards. The CCM must also provide a culturally sensitive and compassionate approach. Despite acting in good faith to maintain professionalism and provide excellent care, a certified case manager may face legal action. In a malpractice suit, it must be proven that the clinician was negligent in their actions and that negligence did cause harm to the client.

As previously discussed in the case-recording section, the CCM's best defense against malpractice is an accurate case file. It is vital to remember that the case file can serve as a legal document and is permissible as evidence in court proceedings. Since the majority of litigants do not seek legal recourse immediately, the CCM must not hope to rely upon their memory. As a licensed practitioner, the certified case manager should consider the following issues: lack of informed consent, breach of confidentiality, negligent referral, bad faith, and premature discharge. Unless it is documented thoroughly in the client's case record, an intervention strategy is not considered complete. Any pertinent information left out of the case file may be perceived as an actual gap in care and possible evidence of negligence.

Without informed consent, a client cannot agree to treatment. Even if a client has signed consent forms upon entry into the hospital, it is also vital that the CCM obtain separate consent for ongoing services post discharge. This is particularly important for working with clients who may not be capable of providing informed consent. For clients suffering from a TBI, the CCM must make note of the consequences of that injury, especially affected brain functions.

If the capacity to fully comprehend the advantages and disadvantages of their treatment is compromised, the patient's attorney, spouse or domestic partner, eldest child, or legal next of kin can be consulted. Unfortunately, this may then lead to the breach of confidentiality for that client. A breach of confidentiality occurs when a clinician provides protected health information that somehow causes harm to the client. If the client is unaware of the potential release of protected health information, even for the continuity of their care, the client may seek legal action. For this reason, it is crucial that the CCM completely disclose the scope of their practice and situations in which they will need to disclose the client's medical information.

For professional and practical purposes, the CCM must be aware of the fact that bad faith is characterized as "consciously doing wrong." Since the CCM is working in collaboration with the patient, insurer, and employer, all interests must be protected. The three components of bad faith include denial of benefits without proper explanation or cause, the clinician's awareness that the denial is erroneous, and improper administration of claims processing once the appeal is filed. If the CCM must issue a denial of benefits while acting in accordance with the dictates of the insurer, it is bad faith for the case manager to issue that denial without proper cause. The bad faith continues if the clinician does not attempt to provide the client with the necessary information to appeal the denial. If the client is able to provide evidence of improper behavior, the CCM may face civil or criminal charges, or experience a temporary or permanent loss of licensure.

Privacy and Confidentiality

Throughout their work with patients, CCMs must uphold the strictest level of confidentiality. As previously stated in the case recording section, the CCM must guard the client's medical records. Unfortunately, the case manager is not the only individual with access to the medical records. Administrative support staff, physicians and nurses, government agencies, and other members of the interdisciplinary team will require access. The Health Insurance Portability and Accountability Act (HIPAA) provides the CCM with the parameters to guard against unlawful or unnecessary use and release of medical information. Whether paper documents, prescriptions, diagnoses, treatment plans, or electronic records are in question, HIPAA regulations require that the prudent clinician exercise extreme caution regarding their release.

Compliance with an organization-wide privacy policy is of paramount importance. Each individual with the potential to come into contact with protected health information must be advised of the privacy policy. The clinician must act as the gatekeeper, providing the information about any particular client's case to those specifically entitled to the information.

The rule of thumb to maintain the secured control of access to medical records is to provide that information on a need-to-know basis. The need-to-know rule refers to individuals who must view the client's protected health information for the sole purpose of providing care. These individuals are to have access to the minimum amount of information necessary to perform the task at hand, nothing more. Only the minimum amount of information required to complete the tasks of caring for the patient should ever be released. Signed, dated, and witnessed informed-consent forms that outline the types of information that can be released must be a mandatory facet of any treatment plan.

Paper documents must be stored under lock and key with access only to the CCM and necessary staff. Destruction of paper documents must occur through the shredding of those documents, or professionals proficient in document destruction can be enlisted for larger organizations. For electronic files and reports, the clinician must be diligent in the security of their desktop and the actual computer through the use of computer screen locks, shortened time-out locks, or black-out screens whenever the computer is left unattended. Computer access must also be limited. The clinician should consider placing the computer behind locked doors, with passwords that are changed frequently, multiple firewalls, and careful screening of incoming emails and documents to guard against computer viruses.

Whenever possible, electronic transfers of medical information, including emails and faxes, must be sent securely. The most effective process is to verbally confirm that the fax number is correct and stored in a secure location away from those without a need to know. Again, limit information to the individuals who must have the information to perform their jobs.

Finally, any transmission of electronic medical records must contain a basic disclaimer advising the recipient on how to proceed if the documents were received in error, such as:

- This communication contains confidential information.

- If you have received this information in error, please notify the sender immediately by phone and return the original to the address listed on the form.

- Any distribution or reproduction of this transmission by anyone other than the intended party is strictly prohibited.

That verbiage, or something similar to it, should be added to all documents, emails, and other transmitted medical records. The role adopted by the clinician in this instance is as a gatekeeper, ensuring that only the correct individuals receive the necessary information.

Risk Management

Inherent in all types of work environments is some degree of occupational hazard. From retail to construction, to the medical or corporate realms, each cross section must develop a plan of action to prevent workplace injuries. **Risk management** is the process of identifying actual and potential hazards and developing cost-effective and efficient strategies to prevent their occurrence. A **sentinel event** can be described as an adverse incident that has led to, or has the potential to lead to, a catastrophic outcome, requiring an immediate intervention. The CCM is often utilized during a postmortem examination of a sentinel event or near miss, in order to help establish a comprehensive plan to prevent the incidence of future injuries. In this instance, the clinician is acting as a communicator, navigator, collaborator, and advocate.

Immediately after any workplace accident or near miss, it is necessary to complete an **incident report**. Within this report are the variables that contributed to the problem. Individuals involved are interviewed, the scene is examined, and management is notified. The CCM reviewing the incident report is generally looking for the following information: Who was involved? What happened? When did it happen? Where did it happen? Why did it happen? How did it happen?

Acting as the investigator, the clinician starts at the beginning. The "who" refers to the specific employees involved, who may also be seeking benefit coverage. The "what" refers to the incident itself. Describing what happened in as much detail as possible will help guide later concerns of how to implement proposed changes. When the incident occurred is equally important. If the incident occurred during peak business hours, after normal business hours, during approved overtime, or during inclement weather, the "when" plays a role in managing future risks. The "where" of the incident is the exact location of the occurrence. Did the event occur in the office, adjacent or nonessential work areas, parking garage, elevator, etc.? The "why," however, is one of the most crucial aspects of this investigation. Why refers to whether or not proper procedures and policies were followed, which may directly impact liability in many workplace-injury cases.

Finally, the "how" is the most necessary question to answer. How the incident occurred refers to three main possibilities. Was the incident precipitated by: **human error**, such as operating the machinery while overtired or wearing improper clothing; **technical error**, such as malfunctioning or poorly maintained equipment; or **procedural error**, like failing to adhere to proper procedures? The answers to each of these questions will guide the CCM and the rest of the risk-management team to the next step in the process, which is the root-cause analysis.

During the **root-cause analysis**, the risk-management team will utilize the answers gleaned from the incident reports and interviews to determine the main cause of the sentinel event. Changing the focus from the problem to the solution, the CCM will act as the collaborator with the risk-management team to move into a dialogue regarding the gaps in procedures, policies, workforce, and/or environment that need to be addressed. The primary objective is to prevent future occurrences of a similar nature, while preserving the factors that did not contribute to the problem. The best changes to implement are feasible, efficient, and cost effective. Once it is confirmed which changes will be made and the management team agrees with the proposal, the policies are changed as needed and the workforce is informed. Acting as the communicator, the CCM may be asked to contribute the memorandum prepared for company-wide distribution.

Depending on the type of event and related injuries, the risk management process can take hours, weeks, or months to be completed.

Self-Care and Well-Being as a Professional

The CCM is tasked with the responsibility to ensure that their patients receive timely, effective, and appropriate care at all times. The expectation is that the CCM enlists and exhausts all available resource services in an effort to guarantee the interventions provided are uninterrupted, detailed, and personalized for each patient they encounter. The CCM, acting as the single point of contact for the family and caregivers, must periodically support their needs for respite. For clients with profound disability, respite may be required more often for their caregivers. Patients are encouraged to consider their emotional needs as well. Conversely, the CCM must utilize those same skills to care for themselves.

It is crucial that the CCM creates an atmosphere of self-acceptance, empathy, and compassion when working with their patients. This cannot be accomplished if the CCM is overtired, functioning on little sleep, or neglects his or her own needs. In order to model these capabilities, the CCM must first possess them. Time away from work (TAFW) and preplanned time off (PPTO) are essential. Ideally, the best option is to remove oneself from the work environment completely. Eliminating access to voicemail, email, or patient's files will prevent any opportunity for distraction from the goal of relaxing. This further illustrates the importance of maintaining accurate records, so that alternate clinicians may follow up with the cases that require attention.

Repeated daily immersion in their caseloads and resolving the problems of patients affected by trauma can be emotionally draining. This prolonged interaction with clients in their weakest state can also be physically taxing and may lead to caregiver burnout. The old adage is true: You cannot drink from an empty cup. It is crucial that the CCM develop strategies to detect caregiver burnout early and address it quickly. Simple, self-care activities like practicing proper nutrition, meditation, journaling, exercise, or spending time with family and friends can "recharge" the batteries.

Another crucial aspect of self-care can include psychotherapy, religious counseling, and/or support groups for mental health professionals. All of these environments respect the confidentiality of the client and normalize the feelings that the CCM may have that are typically associated with caregiver burnout. The majority of mental health professionals acknowledge the need to receive concurrent therapy themselves. It is inevitable that work with clients in various stages of recovery, with different reactions and emotional states, may trigger feelings in the clinician that need to be addressed. These groups also help to delineate the line between personal and professional responsibilities. The comradery of the group dynamic can serve as a forum to receive positive feedback as a practitioner, not consulting on individual cases. Each clinician may be encouraged to highlight times in their work with anonymous clients, providing insight to their colleagues. The group members can hold each other accountable for lapses in self-care while maintaining appropriate boundaries. Overall, any legal activity that creates a safe space to relax and release the tensions of the workday are acceptable.

Standards of Practice

The certified case manager plays numerous roles throughout the life of any case. **The Case Management Society of America** (CMSA) governs the scope of practice for the CCM. Whether acting as the collaborator, advocate, manager, communicator, professional, or navigator, the goal is always to achieve the best possible outcome for all parties involved. These guiding principles of practice empower the client to achieve the best possible outcomes. Although each role has a specific purpose, the CCM utilizes them interchangeably, often taking on several roles at once.

Acting as the collaborator and professional, the clinician works together with the client, their family, and appropriate health care providers to create and execute the plan of care. During the initial portion of any case, the CCM remains aware of the need to join forces with multiple providers to assess the plan of care periodically and make adjustments in the treatment plan as needed.

Next, the CCM takes on the roles of advocate and expert. Following evidence-based standards of care, the clinician is able to guide the client toward traditional and nontraditional options regarding their treatment. Once an informed decision is made, the plan is followed. The adoption of the role as the expert moves the CCM to take the initiative to present the client with the typical results of each intervention.

When the clinician acts as the manager, their role is to merely supervise the situation, stepping up only as the situation requires them to do so. Empowering the client to self-determine the results of treatment whenever it is feasible engenders a sense of trust and rebuilds the client's confidence in themselves.

Applying the appropriate legal and federal legislations and basic employer insurance coverage to obtain payment for the necessary services is also crucial. Here, the CCM returns to the roles of expert and navigator by sifting through the numerous applicable options and locating the most efficient and cost-effective options for long-term results.

Practice Questions

1. What is the primary goal of the PPACA?
   a. To provide American citizens with appropriate and affordable medical coverage.
   b. To ensure that insurance companies are penalized for providing high-cost insurance.
   c. To prevent discrimination against individuals without health insurance.
   d. To provide basic essential health benefits to all children in the United States.

2. Why is it important to obtain informed consent from a client?
   a. To ensure that the CCM is paid for services rendered.
   b. To make sure that the CCM cannot be sued for malpractice.
   c. To confirm that the client was advised of all of the aspects of the treatment plan.
   d. To confirm that the correct providers were enlisted for the client's treatment.

3. Which of the following is NOT an acceptable way to secure protected information in client files?
   a. Shredding nonessential patient information whenever necessary.
   b. Utilizing a Document Management System (DMS).
   c. Keeping copies of all client information in the home office of the CCM.
   d. Providing information only to those who need to know.

4. Which statement best describes the concept of veracity?
   a. Providing compassionate care to every client.
   b. Practicing in an ethically sound manner.
   c. Providing options to the client that are grounded in truth.
   d. Taking the vow to do no harm to any patient.

5. What is the purpose of COBRA?
   a. To increase vocational training for individuals with disabilities.
   b. To allow the family members of disabled persons to take an unpaid leave to care for them.
   c. To strictly prohibit discrimination against persons with disabilities.
   d. To allow individuals to maintain employer medical benefits in the event of loss of employment.

6. Robert is a patient that has sustained an injury that requires the transfusion of blood products in order to preserve his life. Robert is a Jehovah's Witness, and his religion does not allow for allogenic blood transfusion. How should the CCM proceed?
   a. Check to see if any advance directives have been signed, and if they explicitly deny allogenic blood transfusions. If not, proceed with the transfusion without the client's knowledge.
   b. Contact the affiliated clergy and ask them to tell the client to receive the transfusion.
   c. Decline to continue as this is in direct conflict with the standard of practice for the CCM to "do no harm."
   d. Discuss the client's concerns and review alternatives with the hematologist.

7. Maria has sustained a crushing injury and is in a drug-induced coma. The physicians have deemed the client is near death and will remain on life support indefinitely. The client's next of kin, her husband, is adamant that his wife would not want to remain on life support. Which is the BEST response for the CCM?

a. Contact the affiliated clergy and ask them to discuss the matter with the family.

b. Decline to continue as this is in direct conflict with the standard of practice for the CCM to "do no harm."

c. Check to see if any advance directives have been signed, and if they explicitly deny any life-saving measures, proceed according to the client's final wishes.

d. Allow the client's husband to make the final decision regarding the cessation of life support.

8. Which statement explains BEST why it is important to maintain accurate case files?

a. To make sure that the CCM cannot be sued for malpractice.

b. To maintain an accurate, chronological timeline of the plan of care.

c. To ensure that the CCM is paid for services rendered.

d. To confirm that the client was advised of all of the aspects of the treatment plan.

9. Regarding "meaningful use," which statement BEST explains how the CCM demonstrates compliance?

a. Providing evidence that all client records are not only properly secured and that their privacy has been protected, but that the CCM has the appropriate credentials.

b. Creating not only a clearinghouse of information that all providers can access, but also a formula that requires those providers to verify that the use of the database results in improved outcomes for patients.

c. Providing evidence that the CCM has met the standards of practice in working with clients and that all client records are properly secured and their privacy has been protected.

d. Producing records for the supervision received during each case to show the CCM has provided care.

10. What is NOT considered a "bad faith" action by the CCM?

a. The improper administration of administrative denials of benefits.

b. Failure of the CCM to explain the denial of benefits.

c. The client's awareness of the erroneous denial of benefits.

d. Personality conflicts between the client and CCM.

11. Which is the BEST statement that should be added to all electronic transmissions of client records?

a. This communication contains confidential information. If you have received this document in error, please forward to the correct individual. No additional action is needed.

b. This communication contains confidential information. This document must be shredded immediately if you are not the intended recipient. No additional action is needed.

c. This communication contains confidential information. If you have received this information in error, please notify the sender by phone and return the original to the address listed on the form. Any distribution or reproduction of this transmission by anyone other than the intended party is strictly prohibited.

d. None of the above.

12. Eduardo works in a meat-packing plant and recently sustained an injury that resulted in his hand being mangled and later amputated. The client is the meat-packing company and has enlisted the CCM to conduct a root-cause analysis to determine the cause of the accident. What is the primary goal of the CCM in this situation?

    a. The CCM must ensure that there are no grounds for the employee to receive medical coverage.

    b. The CCM must prove that the employee is at fault in the incident.

    c. The CCM must determine the cause of the incident in order to prevent any future incidents.

    d. The CCM must contact legal authorities to investigate the plant's procedures.

13. Which of the following statements BEST explains the primary objective of a root-cause analysis?

    a. To prevent future occurrences of a similar nature, while preserving the factors that did not contribute to the problem.

    b. To discredit and deny the medical claim of the client.

    c. To save the company from future financial loss.

    d. None of the above.

14. Which statement is the BEST response for how the CCM should counsel a family member or caregiver experiencing burnout?

    a. The CCM should counsel the caregiver to permanently institutionalize the client.

    b. The caregiver should be advised to consider antidepressant or anxiety medications.

    c. The CCM should encourage the caregiver to consider respite care.

    d. The caregiver should be counseled to consider therapy.

15. Which statement BEST explains a scenario in which a client has the capacity to consent to treatment?

    a. A client suffering from a condition impairing the function of the mind or brain.

    b. An individual that is unable to understand, retain, and weigh the relevant information provided.

    c. A client who is unable to communicate a decision.

    d. A client suffering from a condition impairing the visual field.

16. What is the BEST preparation for a CCM who has been asked to appear for a deposition regarding the outcome of one of their cases?

    a. Seek legal counsel immediately to determine how to respond.

    b. Confer with colleagues to find out what they would do.

    c. Contact the client to determine the reason for the lawsuit.

    d. Review the client's case files to uncover any areas of concern.

17. What is the BEST explanation of why self-care is important for the CCM?

    a. To model appropriate self-care to clients and caregivers.

    b. In order to better connect with clients and their families.

    c. To preserve their own personal mental health.

    d. None of the above.

18. Brittany is receiving case management regarding a workplace injury that resulted in a below-the-knee amputation. The client received the notification of the denial to her post office box approximately eight weeks earlier and is not sure how to proceed. Under the ERISA laws, what is the BEST response for the CCM in this situation?

a. The case manager must review the denial letter for the actual date in order to determine if the legal appeal time has passed.

b. The case manager must advise the client that the employer is responsible for approving the claim, no matter the circumstance.

c. The case manager must call the insurance company to file an appeal on the client's behalf immediately.

d. The case manager must advise the client that filing an appeal will be unsuccessful and that there is no need to do so.

19. What entity governs the standards of practice for the CCM?

a. The National Society of Case Management.

b. The National Association of Social Workers.

c. The American Nurses Association.

d. The Case Management Society of America.

20. Josephine has been receiving case management due to an injury sustained during a bus versus pedestrian accident. Josephine was the bus driver and sustained a TBI after unsuccessfully turning to avoid the pedestrian. Although it was determined that the brakes on the bus malfunctioned and Josephine was not at fault, she continues to suffer from PTSD along with residual symptoms from the temporal-lobe TBI. Josephine's husband Andrew was the initial caregiver, but filed for divorce after six months, as he was unable to handle caring for his wife. As the spouse, Andrew was legally entitled to receive periodic progress reports, and did often request them. One year later, after a particularly difficult session in OT, Josephine responded with extreme frustration and stormed out of treatment crying and yelling that the treatment plan was moving too fast. Andrew called the CCM to ask the CCM what had occurred during the treatment, stating that Josephine was inconsolable. Andrew calls the CCM and is demanding to review the current treatment plan for Josephine immediately or the CCM will face legal action for malpractice. Which statement below is the BEST response without breaking the patient's confidentiality?

a. Hang up the phone, as any information provided is a violation of the client's privacy.

b. Review the client's file to determine if the advance directive is current and includes Andrew.

c. Contact the client to obtain consent to speak with the estranged spouse.

d. Request that the estranged spouse and client come in together to discuss the client's case.

21. Which of the following questions is NOT typically a part of the immediate investigation following a sentinel event?

a. Who was directly involved with the incident in question?

b. When did the actual incident occur?

c. What can be done to prevent a similar incident from occurring?

d. How exactly did the actual incident occur?

Answer Explanations

1. A: The PPACA was created to ensure that all Americans receive essential medical benefits at an affordable rate. Choice *B* is incorrect. Although specific sanctions are levied against insurance companies that fail to comply, this is not the goal of the act. Choice *C* is incorrect. Discrimination is strictly prohibited against persons without health coverage, and this legislation does address that issue by providing health coverage. This is not, however, the primary goal of the act. Choice *D* is incorrect. Although the PPACA is providing essential health benefits to children, that is not the focus of this legislation.

2. C: This answer is correct. It is crucial that the client's awareness of the plan of care be confirmed in writing. Choice *A* is incorrect. Although the fee schedule is also negotiated with the client and the cost of services both with and without CCM intervention must be presented (if applicable), the informed consent is for treatment purposes, not for payment. Choice *B* is incorrect. The CCM can be sued for malpractice for any reason. The presence of a signed consent form does not prevent the CCM from facing legal action. Choice *D* is incorrect. Although this information is included in the client's case file, the actual informed consent document must include the client's awareness of the plan of care.

3. C: This answer is correct. Files may be kept in a separate location, but must always be secured under lock and key. Choice *A* is incorrect because any nonessential paper documents must be shredded whenever possible. Choice *B* is incorrect. The DMS's are designed to protect patient information. Choice *D* is incorrect. It is the best practice to provide protected health information only to those that need to know in order to continue the care of the client.

4. C: This answer is correct. The CCM must ensure that interventions are truthful and presented plainly. There must be no use of jargon, technical language, or unnecessary information. Choice *A* is incorrect. Although it is always appropriate to maintain a sense of compassion while caring for clients, this is not the formal definition of veracity. Choice *B* is incorrect. Ethical treatment is a tenant of the basic standards of practice for all CCM's, but this is not the formal definition of veracity. Choice *D* is incorrect. Every clinician must ensure that their interventions do not bring harm to their clients, but this is not the formal definition of veracity.

5. D: This answer is correct. Specifically related to rehabilitation, this act allows for the employee, spouse, or dependent children to continue to receive medical coverage for a minimum of eighteen months and a maximum of thirty-six months. Choice *A* is incorrect. This response describes the Workforce Innovation and Opportunity Act of 2014. Choice *B* is incorrect. This describes the Family Medical Leave Act of 1993. Choice *C* is incorrect. This is the purpose of the Americans With Disabilities Act of 1990.

6. D: This answer is correct. It is always appropriate to utilize the physicians when presenting the options for treatment. Doing this will ensure that the client has the correct information to choose their preferred treatment. Choice A is incorrect. This is a violation of the client's rights. If the client is lucid and able to provide informed consent, the CCM cannot override the client's decisions. Choice B is incorrect. Although it is a good idea to contact the affiliated clergy of the client's religion for support, the decision is to be left to the client as to the proper course of treatment. Choice C is incorrect. It is unethical to abandon a client during treatment unless there is an emergent and unavoidable need to do so. The CCM must adhere to the client's wishes, even if the CCM does not agree.

7. C: This answer is correct. It is incumbent upon the CCM to locate any advance directives to confirm the patient's final wishes and ensure that they are followed. Choice *A* is incorrect. Although this is an appropriate response, this is not the best answer. The CCM must take the lead on this case and attempt to confirm the client's wishes. Choice *B* is incorrect. The CCM cannot abandon a client during a case simply due to the client's decision not to pursue the options presented by the clinician. Choice *D* is incorrect. The appropriate action would be to first check for any advance directives and follow them if they do exist.

8. B: This answer is correct. Case files must be accurate in order to confirm the exact treatment plan agreed upon by the client. Choice *A* is incorrect. The maintenance of accurate case files cannot prevent the CCM from facing a lawsuit. Choice *C* is incorrect. The maintenance of accurate files does not guarantee payment for services. Choice *D* is incorrect. Although this is correct, it is not the best answer. Case files must be accurate in order to confirm the exact treatment plan agreed upon by the client.

9. B: This answer is correct. The meaningful-use clause requires all providers to show that their work is both appropriate and impactful. Choice *A* is incorrect. Meaningful use does not directly refer to the confidentiality of client files. Choice *C* is incorrect. This is not a definition of meaningful use. Choice *D* is incorrect. Meaningful use does not refer to supervision received by the CCM.

10. D: This answer is correct. Although the rapport between the client and CCM is crucial to the process, it is not necessary for the client and CCM to be friends in order for the treatment plan to succeed. Choice *A* incorrect. Bad faith involves the improper administration of administrative denials of benefits. Choice *B* is incorrect. Bad faith also involves the failure of the CCM to explain the denial of benefits. Choice *C* is incorrect. This is the third and final aspect of bad faith.

11. C: This answer is correct. All of the language in this answer provides specific instruction as to how the document must be handled. Choice *A* is incorrect. The document cannot be forwarded by a third party; this is a violation of HIPAA. Choice *B* is incorrect. The CCM cannot guarantee that the documents have been shredded. It is imperative that the correct fax number be confirmed prior to sending the transmission. Choice *D* is incorrect.

12. C: This answer is correct. The case manager is tasked with investigating the incident to operationalize the best way to prevent a recurrence. Choice A is incorrect. The CCM is not to act in an unethical way. Choice *B* is incorrect. The CCM has not been enlisted to find any party to be at fault, but to determine the root cause of the incident. Choice D is incorrect. Through a systematic investigation, the CCM will be able to determine the cause of the incident and identify all contributing and noncontributing factors.

13. A: This answer is correct. The CCM must seek to determine the primary cause of the incident and all contributing factors in order to enact any necessary policy or procedural changes. Choice *B* is incorrect. The CCM may be acting as an agent of the company, but the primary goal is to prevent future accidents of a similar nature. Choice *C* is incorrect. Although implementing the necessary policy or procedural changes will result in little or no financial loss for the company, this is only as a result of the prevention of similar incidents. Choice *D* is incorrect.

14. C: This answer is correct. It is important for the CCM to remind the caregiver of the importance of caring for themselves just as they do their family member. Choice *A* is incorrect. The decision to admit their ill family member into an institution is a delicate matter. The discussion must also include the client and should not be considered as the only option. Choice *B* is incorrect. Although it may be necessary to consider medications, the medications cannot alleviate any physical stress involved in caring for a family member. Choice *D* is incorrect. This is also a viable option, but is not necessarily going to allow for the caregiver to completely disconnect from their role in order to care for themselves.

15. D: This answer is correct. A client who is blind is still able to hear and comprehend and retain the information presented. That client is also able to weigh the relevant information provided and communicate their decision to consent to treatment. Choice *A* is incorrect. A client unable to utilize their mind cannot form the rational thought required to think clearly. Choice *B* is incorrect. This client would not be able to appreciate the differences between the options presented and would not be able to provide an informed consent. Choice *C* is incorrect. The client in this situation may be able to hear the information, but is unable to respond to communicate that understanding; therefore, they cannot consent.

16. A: This answer is correct. The CCM must immediately consult an attorney to determine the best course of action. Choice *B* is incorrect. Although it is tempting to discuss the case with a colleague, this has the potential to violate the clients' privacy. Choice *C* is incorrect. The CCM is never contacted by the client but is usually served notice of the lawsuit. Contacting the client may only serve to escalate the situation and lead to professional sanctions. Choice *D* is incorrect. Although this is necessary to do, the first response must be to seek legal counsel. The case file will then be pulled and reviewed once the attorney can determine the best course of action.

17. C: This answer is correct. The CCM must work diligently to guard their own well-being in order to provide appropriate care to clients. Choice *A* is incorrect. Although it is important for the CCM to model appropriate self-care, the most important reason is to preserve the well-being of the clinician. Choice *B* is incorrect. This is one of the results of the CCM making self-care a priority. As the CCM effectively manages stress, the CCM is better able to empathize with their clients. Choice *D* is incorrect.

18. A: This answer is correct. According to ERISA, an appeal can be filed if the sixty-day time frame has not expired. Choice *B* is incorrect. Under the ERISA guidelines, the employer does not have to honor an appeal received after the sixty-day time frame has expired. Choice *C* is incorrect. According to ERISA, all appeals must be received in writing. Choice *D* is incorrect. An appeal can be filed if the sixty-day time frame has not expired.

19. D: This answer is correct. Case managers adhere to the practice standards of the CMSA. Choice *A* is incorrect. This entity is fictional. Choice *B* is incorrect. This entity governs the standards of practice for social workers only. Choice *C* is incorrect. This entity governs the standards of practice for nurses only.

20. B: This answer is correct. Prior to disclosing any protected information, the client must either obtain a release of information to do so, or determine if one already exists. If none exists or it has expired, the CCM cannot reveal any information to a third party. Choice *A* is incorrect. It is not a violation of the client's privacy to respond to the caller. The CCM is not allowed, however, to confirm or deny the names and/or treatment plans of clients. Choice *C* is incorrect. A client with a TBI is unable to provide informed consent to sign a release of information or an advance directive. Choice *D* is incorrect. A client with a TBI is unable to provide informed consent to sign a release of information or an advance directive.

21. C: This answer is correct. This question is asked later in the investigation, during the root-cause analysis. The purpose of this question is to determine how to solve the problems gleaned from the initial investigation. Choice *A* is incorrect. This is one of the initial questions asked during the post mortem of a sentinel event. Finding out who was involved will guide who the investigator must interview. Choice *B* is incorrect. This question is also integral to the investigation of the sentinel event. The answer to this question will direct the investigator to any physical cause of the incident. Choice *D* is incorrect. The answer to this question will determine if a human error, mechanical error, or procedural error was the likely cause of the incident.

Index

Dear CCM Certification Test Taker,

We would like to start by thanking you for purchasing this study guide for your CCM Certification exam. We hope that we exceeded your expectations.

Our goal in creating this study guide was to cover all of the topics that you will see on the test. We also strove to make our practice questions as similar as possible to what you will encounter on test day. With that being said, if you found something that you feel was not up to your standards, please send us an email and let us know.

We have study guides in a wide variety of fields. If you're interested in one, try searching for it on Amazon or send us an email.

Thanks Again and Happy Testing!
Product Development Team
info@studyguideteam.com

FREE Test Taking Tips DVD Offer

To help us better serve you, we have developed a Test Taking Tips DVD that we would like to give you for FREE. **This DVD covers world-class test taking tips that you can use to be even more successful when you are taking your test.**

All that we ask is that you email us your feedback about your study guide. Please let us know what you thought about it – whether that is good, bad or indifferent.

To get your **FREE Test Taking Tips DVD**, email freedvd@studyguideteam.com with "FREE DVD" in the subject line and the following information in the body of the email:

   a. The title of your study guide.

   b. Your product rating on a scale of 1-5, with 5 being the highest rating.

   c. Your feedback about the study guide. What did you think of it?

   d. Your full name and shipping address to send your free DVD.

If you have any questions or concerns, please don't hesitate to contact us at freedvd@studyguideteam.com.

Thanks again!

Made in the USA
Columbia, SC
23 August 2020